D0250036

WHAT *to* EAT

if YOU HAVE

CANCER

A Guide to Adding Nutritional Therapy to Your Treatment Plan

MAUREEN KEANE, M.S., AND
DANIELLA CHACE, M.S.

CB
CONTEMPORARY BOOKS

Library of Congress Cataloging-in-Publication Data

Keane, Maureen.
    What to eat if you have cancer: a guide to adding nutritional therapy
to your treatment plan / Maureen Keane and Daniella Chace.
        p.   cm.
    Includes index.
    ISBN 0-8092-3261-8
    1. Cancer—Diet therapy.   2. Cancer—Nutritional aspects.
I. Chace, Daniella.   II. Title.
RC271.D52K43   1996
616.99'40654—dc20   96-14016
                                                                 CIP

Cover design by Kim Bartko
Cover painting by Charlotte Segal: *Tabernacle* (oil on canvas;
48 inches × 66 inches)

Charlotte Segal is an instructor at the International Academy
of Design Chicago and a twenty-one-year cancer survivor.
Segal's paintings and prints are part of numerous corporate
and private collections. "Making art is my way to live beyond
the years God has granted me. I feel I have survived through
sheer will. Further, I view being able to create art as a gift to
be treasured."

Healing Legacies is an arts registry that contains work by
women and men who have experienced breast cancer.
Created in 1993, the registry now represents more than 100
artists and contains more than 500 pieces of visual and
written work. For more information about Healing Legacies,
contact the Breast Cancer Action Group, PO Box 5605,
Burlington, VT 05402. Artists wishing a prospectus should
send a SASE.

Published by Contemporary Books
An imprint of NTC/Contemporary Publishing Company
4255 West Touhy Avenue, Lincolnwood (Chicago), Illinois 60646-1975 U.S.A.
Copyright © 1996 by Maureen Keane and Daniella Chace.
All rights reserved. No part of this book may be reproduced, stored in a retrieval
system, or transmitted in any form or by any means, electronic, mechanical,
photocopying, recording, or otherwise, without the prior permission of
NTC/Contemporary Publishing Company.
Manufactured in the United States of America
International Standard Book Number: 0-8092-3261-8
18   17   16   15   14   13   12   11   10   9   8   7   6   5   4   3

This book is dedicated to the memory of
Michael J. O'Malley, who died unexpectedly on
Valentine's Day, 1996. A gentle giant of an Irishman,
Mike was known for his generous heart and willing hands.
His death has left a hole in all of us who loved him.

Contents

Part II: Friendly Fire: The Nutritional Side Effects of Treatment

Part III: Diet Plans: Developing Your Nutritional Therapy Regime

Part IV: Appendixes

Foreword

*T*he complex problems related to cancer continue to confound physicians and scientists, and, with the exception of lung cancer, the etiology of most malignancies is unknown. We have, however, discovered useful clues regarding the causes of cancer from population studies and epidemiological research. For example, developing countries do not suffer the cancer rates of modern society. The American cancer epidemic is linked to air and water pollution, food-chain contamination, food-processing techniques, smoking, drugs, constant stress (distress), obesity, and a sedentary lifestyle. All of these factors may be connected to cancer causation through nutritional imbalance. It is a recognized fact that two out of three women with breast cancer are obese. Nutritional status is affected by lifestyle choices and dietary habits. Our nutritional status either weakens us, promoting the development of cancer, or strengthens our bodies' defense mechanisms, enhancing our ability to prevent and/or control neoplastic processes.

Epidemiological studies and research into dietary habits suggest that specific, naturally occurring chemicals offer protection against cancer. Science has advanced in the realm of nutrition to a point where we can treat physiological imbalances with specific foods and related substances. For example, food components (antioxidants) may aid and strengthen the immune mechanism, and elements such as fiber may protect against the development of cancer. This publication may enlighten the cancer patient with information that is of extreme value in understanding the cancer process and the treatment thereof. During the last 25 years, many patients under my care have questioned what they can do to change their lifestyles and enhance their ability to prevent and/or cure their malignancy. The information provided herein may prove extremely valuable in answering these queries.

These dietary protocols are suitable for patients at any stage of treatment. A change in lifestyle, including improved nutrition, may enhance traditional cancer therapy. This book defines a program of nutrition as an adjunct to medical cancer therapy. Improved dietary habits and an altered lifestyle may provide powerful support to conventional cancer treatments and, ultimately, the healing process. In the past, many cancer victims have found themselves involved in programs that do not approach the problem in a global, comprehensive manner. Those individuals who take an active, positive role in their treatment may enhance their chance of recovery and a complete cure.

John A. Lung, M.D., cancer surgeon
Mountain States Tumor Institute, Boise, Idaho

Acknowledgments

*W*e would like to thank Dr. Joe Pizzorno, Dr. Jay Littel, Dr. Deb Brammer, Dr. Allan Gaby, and Dr. John Lung for sharing their knowledge with us; Darren and Tonja Hill for contributing their firsthand experiences and hard-earned lessons; David Stevenson for his illustrations; Nels Moulton for his software support; and Merrilee Gomez.

Maureen wishes to thank her husband, John, for his love and support through her cancer treatment, surgery, and recovery; her son, Micheál, for his computer expertise in helping to prepare this manuscript; and her feline accomplice, Maeve, for her constant companionship and unsolicited advice.

Introduction

*I*f you have been diagnosed with cancer, you remember with crystal clarity the moment you got the news. I will never forget.

It all started seventeen years ago on what appeared to be just another day. I was four months pregnant with my second child, and bending over was already difficult. Somehow I was sure this one was going to be a girl. My rough-and-tumble son was eighteen months old, and I was ready for a change. Toddler in tow, I had taken to window shopping for baby clothes. Little-girl clothes with bows and lace.

That day I bent to get a saucepan out of the lower cupboard. Cramps shot through my back, and as I stopped to catch my breath, I could feel the flow of warm blood. Two weeks and two ultrasounds later, we knew the baby had died. But the placenta hadn't; it was still alive and growing. Ten days after the D & C to remove the placenta and fetal remains, my gynecologist phoned. He wanted to see my husband and me in his office immediately. When I asked what was wrong, he simply said he had to discuss the pathology report on the D & C, and it was difficult to discuss "this type of thing" over the phone. I croaked out, "This isn't cancer, is it?" Pause. I've always hated pauses. "No, it isn't cancer." I could almost see him searching for the right words. "But it is something that can become cancer, if it persists. But the D & C probably removed all of it."

A year later I was in an oncologist's office at the University of Washington. That something had apparently persisted. The placental cells of my dead baby were wandering my body, looking for a new home. But no need to worry, I was assured, they probably had spread only into the uterine wall. Chemotherapy should work; it almost always did.

After a CAT scan showed my lungs were clear, I began my first course of chemo with methotrexate. As I tried to get my mind off the needle the nurse was trying without success to stick into the back of my hand, I asked her, "If this disease spreads like cancer and it's treated like cancer, what makes it different from cancer?" She looked up into my eyes and then down again to work on my vein. "When it spreads like this," she said to my hand, "it is cancer." "Oh," was my only reply.

Somehow my first emotion was one of embarrassment. How could I have cancer and not know it? Why hadn't anyone bothered to tell me? *Of course, dummy,* I told myself, *you are seeing an oncologist in an oncology clinic being treated with chemotherapy by an oncology nurse. What did you think you had? But not cancer, not me.* I don't know what was worse those first few weeks: the side effects of the methotrexate or the knowledge that I had cancer. The C word. Not me.

Many friends gave me advice; others sent relics, medals, and cards. Everyone was praying. I made a point of going to a luncheon sponsored by the Irish club immediately after the first treatment. I wanted to show my friends that this disease was not going to get me down. It was the start of Irish week, and the committee in charge of the meal served corned beef and fresh horseradish with an Irish coffee chaser. No one had mentioned nutrition.

The first course of methotrexate didn't work. Neither did the second. No problem, the doctor said, the actinomycin will probably work. But the first course of actinomycin didn't work, and then neither did the second. My oncologist was a great communicator: "You have three options," he told my husband and me over the phone. "Do nothing, and I guarantee you'll be dead in a year. We can put you in the hospital in the fall for combination chemotherapy that will make you quite ill. Or you can have surgery." The cells were probably in the uterus. We opted for surgery. I started one last course of chemo and then had my uterus and tubes removed.

That was sixteen years ago. My hair grew back, and it wasn't long before the other symptoms were just a memory. The only thing I have left is the scar from surgery and a strong dislike of horseradish.

Never once during the sixteen months of tests and treatment did any of my doctors, nurses, or other health care workers ever mention nutrition.

They took the "baby and the bathwater" approach to nutrition and cancer. If nutrition could not cure cancer, then nutrition was useless against cancer. Out the window they would toss it all. They did not understand the true nature of nutrition, which is one of help and support. Nutritional therapy helps your immune system to perform its job better while it supports your healthy cells during the stress of cancer treatment.

Therefore, following the advice in this book will not by itself cure you of cancer. Nutrition therapy alone will not cure cancer. But when nutrition therapy is added to your traditional cancer treatment plan, it can increase your chance of cure as well as the quality of your life.

This book is divided into three parts. Part I is a primer on the body, cancer, and nutrition. It will introduce you to the vocabulary of cancer. Please take the time to read it. It will help you communicate with your doctor and make more informed decisions regarding nutrition. As much as we hate to say it, you will soon be the target of dozens of food supplement salespeople, many of whom will be very aggressive and very uneducated about nutrition and cancer. Be prepared for the hype, and then ignore it.

Part II discusses the various nutritional side effects associated with cancer treatment. Each chapter highlights a particular problem, explains what causes it, and suggests solutions and strategies for coping.

Part III contains the meat of the book. There you will find several diet plans. These are designed to provide a high level of nutrition under conditions often experienced by cancer patients, from weight loss to coping with radiation therapy. Along with each diet plan are recommendations for food supplements.

To develop your own personalized nutrition program, choose from Part III the diet that most closely resembles your situation. Then from Part II add the recommendations for any side effects you may be experiencing.

In the back of the book you will find references to help you participate in your treatment plan. These include a glossary; sample formulas to help you buy supplements; lists of resources for information, support, and products; and details about products mentioned in the book.

This is the book I wish I had been given. I sincerely hope it helps you.

You can start on this program today. A quick excursion to the supermarket with a side trip to the health food store is all you need to take control of your health. Do your health care team a favor and join them. Together you have a much better chance at succeeding.

Just a few words of caution: Do *not* take large doses of any vitamin or food supplement without the knowledge of your doctor. Some vitamins can negate the effects of some treatments.

And one last word of advice: Don't listen to well-meaning (or otherwise) friends. Do not think, "If only I had done this or not done that, I would never have gotten cancer." Forget the past, live in the present, and plan for the future. Do not waste precious energy agonizing about things over which you have no control.

Maureen Keane

Part I

The Body, Cancer, and Nutrition

Getting diagnosed with cancer is somewhat similar to taking a crash course in medical school. Within a few months of your diagnosis you will know more about your particular disease, the organ it is growing in, and the research being conducted than your original family doctor does. This self-education is vitally important to your recovery because knowledge is power—power over your disease and power over your treatment. Go to the library and read everything you can find on your particular situation. Start with your local library and work up to the medical library at the closest medical school. Get on the Internet and search the World Wide Web for treatment options and patient discussion groups. Pick up the phone and call knowledgeable friends for information and advice. Join a support group, subscribe to newsletters, and keep reading and questioning. The more you know, the more options you will have.

Part I of this book was written to help you understand the concepts behind the words and terminology you will soon be learning. If you have just been diagnosed and know little about biology and cancer, this is the best place to start your education. These chapters simplify the anatomy of the body, the physiology of cancer, and the chemistry of nutrition. They explain how and why nutrition therapy works.

This section is also a good introduction to nutrition and cancer treatment for spouses, family members, caregivers, and health care professionals. It will help them to understand what you are trying to accomplish.

I

The Microscopic World
Inside You

*T*o understand what cancer is and how it is treated, you must first become familiar with the miniature world of the cell. This is perhaps the most important chapter of the book, for the cellular level is where cancer begins and where nutrition exerts its effect. This chapter will help you understand the workings of the bodies of your cell citizens and how they divide when healthy.

Imagine for a minute that your body is a country and its cells are the citizens of your country. You, the president, live in the capitol building, the head. For a nation to be strong and healthy, its citizens must have honest work, proper tools to perform that work, a communication system, a transportation system, food and water, and a method to remove waste and trash. They must be protected from the environment and from attack by enemies from within and from without. With your help, the body is able to provide all of these necessities.

Your cell citizens come in all shapes, sizes, and abilities, and they perform an almost endless variety of jobs. Some inhabit the great cities that are your organs; others prefer to live in the country as far away from the bright lights as possible—in your big toe, for instance. But no matter where it lives, each cell has a purpose, an important job that it performs for the good of that great nation, your body: The United States of John or Jane Doe.

Basic Structure of a Cell

We begin this book with an examination of the average cell citizen. Back in the fifties when I was a child, we were taught that a cell was little more than a bag of water with a nucleus floating inside. I fancied that a cell must resemble a raw egg without the brittle outer shell. I always marveled that I didn't scramble myself.

Today we know that cells are highly structured. The entire cell is filled with a scaffolding in which structures called **organelles** are embedded. Organelles are like tiny versions of your body's organs. Each of them has a specific function, and when these functions are interfered with, the result can affect the entire cell body.

Cells have a "skin" called the **plasma membrane**. Attached to the outer surface of the plasma membrane are many protein molecules. Some of these molecules lie on top of the skin or membrane and serve as name tags, identifying to the outside environment what type of cell it is. Other molecules, called **receptor sites**, are attachment spots for hormones and other molecules, including the **antibodies** that are part of immune system. Some molecules are found in groups of two or four and penetrate all the way through the surface of the membrane. These molecules act as a guarded door, allowing water and other small molecules to enter the cell.

In the center of the cell is its "brain," the **nucleus**. This round body is enclosed in a plasma membrane. It holds the **chromatids**, bodies that contain the encoded instructions for all cellular functions. All cells in the body, with the exception of the red blood cells, have a nucleus. A few types even have more than one.

Extending from the membrane of the nucleus to the membrane of the cell are the **cell fibers**. These are filaments that form a three-dimensional scaffold throughout the cell. Serving as the cell's muscles, they contract and expand, producing movement within the cell and allowing the cell to change shape. Embedded in the cell fibers are the organelles (little organs).

The outer membrane of the cell and the membrane of the nucleus are connected by a network of membrane-lined canals called the **endoplasmic reticulum (ER)**. The ER serves as a transportation tunnel and manufacturing site for proteins. Lining some of the ER canals are the **ribosomes**, small round organelles on top of which new proteins are made.

The protein made in the endoplasmic reticulum is funneled into the **Golgi apparatus**, a series of flat, stacked sacks. The Golgi apparatus manufactures large carbohydrate molecules to combine with the proteins, forming **glycoproteins**. As the sacs fill up, they become more globular. The neatly packaged glycoproteins then migrate toward the cell surface and pass through the cell membrane. Outside the cell, the sacs break open, and their contents are released. These contents can range from mother's milk to digestive juices to sweat.

The energy for these activities and others is manufactured in the **mitochondria**, sausage-shaped organelles composed of two membranes. The outer membrane gives each mitochondrion a smooth appearance. The inner membrane resembles a too-large sausage that has to be folded to fit inside. On top of this folded inner membrane lie as many as 500 enzymes used to produce energy. Mitochondria have their own DNA (genetic material) and their own protein-producing ribosomes. This has led many researchers to speculate they are the descendants of bacteria that were swallowed but never digested by larger cells billions of years ago.

The digestive system of the cell is a collection of **lysosomes**. These are sacs that contain enzymes for digesting all of the major components of a cell. When an object—for example, a bacteria—gets inside of a cell, it is surrounded by a lysosome, which digests the intruder. Lysosomes can also burst and digest the cell they live in. Thus, they are sometimes called "suicide bags."

How Cells Divide

Different types of cells have different life spans, depending on their location and function. Some cells, such as neurons, (the cells of nerves), are made to last a human lifetime. Others, like white blood cells, live for only two days. The cells that line the gastrointestinal tract live only for thirty-six hours before they are sloughed off. And just like people, cells can get sick and injured, causing death. For a tissue to function properly, damaged or dead cells must be replaced.

New cells are produced by the process of cell division, or **mitosis**, during which one parent cell divides into two identical daughter cells. A cell knows when to grow or divide by talking to its neighbors. A cell in a new neighborhood of rapidly growing tissue will get the go-ahead to propagate, while a cell in a crowded healthy tissue will be told more citizens are not welcome. Since a good cell citizen is a team player, it divides or travels only when the community deems it proper and necessary.

Cell division starts inside the nucleus, the cell's "brain." Inside the nucleus lie all of the coded instructions needed for the day-to-day life of the cell. These instructions are in the cell's genetic material, **deoxyribonucleic acid (DNA)**.

A DNA molecule is elegantly simple. Often called the double helix, it resembles a long spiral ladder with one complete turn to every ten rungs. The backbones of the ladder are composed of **deoxyriboses** (a type of sugar) that alternate with **phosphate groups**. The rungs of the ladder are composed of molecules called **bases**. Each rung is composed of base pairs—two bases connected weakly in the center. The base pairs fit together like pieces of a jigsaw puzzle.

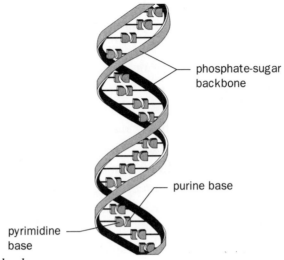

phosphate-sugar
backbone

purine base

pyrimidine
base

DNA molecule

In humans, there are two types of bases. The purine bases, adenine and guanine, are made from the amino acid purine, and the pyrimidine bases, cytosine and thymine, are made from the amino acid pyrimidine. The purine base adenine always pairs with the pyrimidine base thymine and the purine base guanine always pairs with the pyrimidine base cytosine. This means that if you were to look at the rungs in one DNA ladder, they might read adenine-thymine, guanine-cytosine, thymine-adenine. In another DNA molecule, they might read cytosine-guanine, adenine-thymine, cytosine-guanine. The sequence of the three base pairs forms a code word, or **codon**. In this way base pairs are letters, and codons are words. These letters and words form the language of life.

When a cell begins to divide, the DNA molecules coil into rod-shaped bodies called **chromosomes**. Each chromosome makes a duplicate of itself. On a molecular level this is accomplished by pulling the DNA ladder apart by the legs. The rungs separate at the weakest point, between the base pairs. Each half rebuilds into a whole molecule, using free bases floating in the nucleus. On a molecular level, the result is two identical DNA molecules. During the last phase of cell duplication, the cell cytoplasm and cell membrane pinch inward between the two sets of chromosomes, forming two cells.

But not all duplications result in exact duplicates. Base pairs can be lost or placed in a different order. This is called a **mutation**. It results in lost words or sentences, misspelled codon words, or words being out of order in the cellular instructions.

Mutations are not at all rare, but they are often minor and the cell is able to get the gist of the instructions despite the errors. But occasionally a whole section of words is lost or misspelled into gibberish. When this happens to vital cell documents, the mutation causes death.

To prevent this, our cells have developed a backup system. Special enzymes zip up and down the DNA ladders, fixing misspelled words. They're sort of like a DNA spell-checker. But the spell-checker works well only when it is supplied with the enzymes it needs.

Summary

Cells, like people, contain a number of specialized structures. Each structure, or organelle, performs a specific job. The cell's activities are directed by the nucleus, which contains the genetic material. When a cell divides, the genetic material divides. When errors occur in this process, the result is a mutation.

2

Tissues

*C*ancer cells and tumors share many of the characteristics of the tissues from which they originate. Your physician will use many of the terms found in this chapter when describing your tumor. The type of cell the cancer originated from and the type of cells it is growing with determine the type and length of treatment.

Each of your cell citizens belongs to a **tissue**, a community of physically similar cells. Cell citizens of the same tissue type belong to a sort of family or union. They may not live in the same neighborhood or town, but they look alike and perform the same job. There are four main types of tissue: epithelial tissue, connective tissue, muscle tissue, and nervous tissue. Cancers are named after the type of tissue from which they developed, as well as the location of the tumor.

Epithelial Tissue

Most of the cells you can see on your body are **epithelial cells**. Cells in this clan earn their living by covering, lining, secreting, and absorbing. Wherever your body comes into contact with the outside environment, epithelial tissue can be found. It covers all of the external parts of your body from hair to toenails, lines the cavities of body organs, and forms the inner lining of the body cavities. The gastrointestinal tract from mouth to anus is lined with epithelial tissue. So is the respiratory system. The inside of the uterus, bladder, and all blood vessels is lined with epithelial tissue.

There are two kinds of epithelial tissue: glandular and membranous. **Glandular epithelial tissue** contains small

Examples of Malignant Tumors

Carcinomas
(Cancers Originating in the Epithelial Tissue)

TYPE	LOCATION
adenocarcinoma	gland
adenocarcinoma of the lung	lung glandular tissue
gastric adenocarcinoma	stomach glandular epithelium
pancreatic carcinoma	pancreas
papillocarcinoma	epithelial tissue
melanoma	skin

Sarcomas
(Cancers Originating in the Bone and Soft Tissues)

TYPE	LOCATION
fibrosarcoma	fibrous tissue
hemangiosarcoma	blood vessels
chondrosarcoma	cartilage
synovial sarcoma	synovial tissue (lining of the joints)
osteosarcoma	bone
liposarcoma	fat
leiomyosarcoma	smooth muscle
rhabdomyosarcoma	striated muscle

Leukemias
(Malignancies of the Leukocytes, or White Blood Cells)

TYPE	CELL AFFECTED/ORIGIN
acute lymphocytic leukemia (ALL)	lymphocytes
chronic lymphocytic leukemia (CLL)	lymphocytes
acute myelogenous leukemia (AML)	bone marrow
chronic myelogenous leukemia (CML)	bone marrow
chronic lymphoid leukemia (CLL)	lymphoid cells
erythroleukemia	erythrocytic tissue
myelocytic leukemia	granulocytic tissue
reticuloendotheliosis (hairy cell leukemia)	lymphoid cells

Lymphomas
(Connective Tissue Cancers
of the Lymph System)

TYPE	TISSUE AFFECTED
Hodgkin's disease	lymph nodes
malignant granuloma	lymph nodes
lymphogranuloma	lymph nodes

Cancers of the Nervous Tissue
(Named After the Type of Cell
in Which They Occur)

TYPE	LOCATION
glioma	glial tissue
neurilemmic sarcoma	nerve sheaths
astrocytomas	astrocytes (a type of neuroglial cell)
retinoblastoma	retina
meningeal sarcoma	meninges (the membrane that covers the brain)

Other Malignancies

TYPE	TISSUE AFFECTED/TISSUE OF ORIGIN
multiple myeloma	plasma cells and bone marrow
choriocarcinoma	placenta (germ cell tumor)
dysgerminoma	ovary (germ cell tumor)
seminoma	testes (germ cell tumor)
thyoma	thymus

exocrine glands (glands that secrete their products into ducts). These secrete various substances into the environment, organ cavity, or body cavity. In the gastrointestinal tract, for instance, glandular epithelial cells make the passage of food and waste products easier by secreting a lubricating mucus. In the stomach they secrete hydrochloric acid and the intrinsic factor necessary for vitamin B_{12} absorption.

Membranous epithelial tissues serve as coverings or

linings. These cells are classifed according to their shape and type of cell layer.

- Membranous cells come in three shapes. **Squamous** cells are flat and scale-like. **Cuboidal** cells are cube-shaped and have more cytoplasm. **Columnar** cells are taller than they are wide and look like a standing column.
- Membranous cells come in four types of cell layers. **Simple epithelium** is only one layer deep. **Stratified epithelium** is layered one cell on top of another. **Pseudostratified columnar epithelium** gives the appearance of having more than one cell layer but is actually only one layer deep. **Transitional epithelium** is composed of differing cell shapes which are layered.

Put these two classifications together for the various types of membranous epithelial cells. For example, simple squamous epithelium is composed of flat cells one layer deep. Substances easily cross this kind of tissue. Stratified transitional epithelium has the ability to stretch and so lines the bladder.

Epithelial cells are avascular (do not have a blood supply). When they die, they slough off. A good example of this is the gradual shedding of skin cells or the not-so-gradual shedding of dandruff. Cancer cells in epithelial tissue also can shed, making them easy to collect and examine. This is useful for diagnosis, because cancer cells have a very distinctive appearance under the microscope. The familiar Pap smear is a good example of how shed cells can be useful in cancer diagnoses. It is performed by taking a smear of shed uterine cells from the cervix.

Epithelial cells must divide very quickly to replace cells lost to wear and tear. Therefore, cancer treatments (such as chemotherapy and radiation), which target rapidly dividing cancer cells, will also affect epithelial tissue.

Cancerous tumors of the surface epithelium are called **carcinomas**. Those of the glandular epithelium are called **adenocarcinomas**.

Connective Tissue

Connective tissue forms the delicate webs, fluid blood, and hard bones used to connect, support, transport, and defend the body. It is a complex of live cells separated by various types of fibers embedded in a nonliving material called the **matrix** or **ground substance**. The type of matrix material and fiber determines what kind of characteristic the connective tissue exhibits. For example, cartilage tissue has a gellike matrix, bone tissue has a hard mineral matrix, and blood tissue has a liquid matrix.

Connective tissue can be divided into a variety of types, some of which overlap. They include the following:

- Loose ordinary connective or **areolar tissue** connects tissues and organs by acting as a flexible glue. Its matrix is a soft, viscous gel.
- **Adipose connective tissue** resembles areolar tissue with the addition of adipose (fat storage) cells. It forms protective pads around the kidneys and other organs and serves as body insulation.
- **Dense fibrous connective tissue** is made up of a mix of collagen and elastic fibers in a liquid matrix. It forms tendons and ligaments and is also found in the dermal layer of the skin. Scars are made of this type of tissue. It offers a flexible but strong connection between bone and muscle tissues.
- **Reticular tissue** is composed of reticular cells that coat slender, branching reticular fibers forming a three-dimensional network. Reticular tissue forms the scaffold of the spleen, lymph nodes, and thymus and so is an important part of the immune system. The meshlike qualities of this tissue allow the organs to filter harmful substances and cells from the blood and lymph.
- **Bone (osseous) tissue** is made up of osteocytes embedded in a matrix of collagen fibers and mineral salts. The mineral salts give bones their hardness.

- **Cartilage** consists of chondrocytes embedded in a flexible gristlike matrix. Your earlobes contain elastic cartilage, your knee contains fibrocartilage, and your respiratory tubes are held open by rings of hyaline cartilage. Cartilage tissue has no blood supply, so nutrients must diffuse in. For this reason, tears in cartilage do not heal quickly or well.

- **Myeloid tissue** forms the bone marrow and cells derived from it, including the red blood cells and platelets, as well as the granulocytes and monocytes needed for the immune system.

- **Blood tissue** is the most unusual connective tissue. It is in a liquid form and so does not contain any fibers or a ground substance. Blood tissue has two components: the liquid part, called **plasma**, and the solid cellular part, which contains the red blood cells (**erythrocytes**), the platelets, and the white blood cells (**leukocytes**) of the immune system.

Cancers that occur in the bone and the soft tissues (connective and muscle) are called **sarcomas**. Sarcomas are most common in children. Cancers of the lymphatic system are called **lymphomas**. Lymphomas can arise anywhere in the lymph system but most commonly occur in the lymph nodes. **Multiple myeloma** is a cancer of the plasma cells. **Leukemias** are cancers of the blood-forming tissues. Leukemias affect both the ability of the cell to mature and the ability of the cell to perform its function.

Muscle Tissue

Muscle cells are the expert movers of the body. They can be divided into three types:

1. **Skeletal muscle** tissue attaches to bones and moves the skeleton. It is sometimes referred to as "striated muscle" because under a microscope the cell fibers have

cross stripes, or as "voluntary muscle" because you can move it at will.

2. **Visceral muscle** tissue is found in the soft internal organs of the body (the viscera). It is sometimes referred to as "smooth muscle" because of its lack of cross stripes or as "involuntary muscle" because it is not ordinarily controlled by will.

3. **Cardiac muscle** tissue forms the walls of the heart. It is an involuntary muscle with many of the attributes of striated muscle.

Sarcomas of the muscle tissue usually occur in children. Cancer of the striated muscle is the fifth most common cancer in children after leukemias and lymphomas, central nervous system tumors, neuroblastoma, and Wilms' tumor.

Nervous Tissue

Nervous tissue forms the organs of the brain, spinal cord, and nerves. Nerve cells are the telephone and data communication workers of the body. They make electronic communications possible. There are two types of nervous tissue:

1. Nerve cells, or **neurons**, are the cells that actually perform the transmissions. Neurons have a cell body, called the **soma**; one **axon**, which can be as long as one meter; and one or more **dendrites** (nerve fibers).

2. **Neuroglia cells** support and connect the neurons. For example, **Schwann cells** make up the neurilemma and myelin coats of neurons. **Astrocytes** form tight webs around the capillaries in the brain. Together with the capillary walls, they form the **blood-brain barrier**, the stucture responsible for keeping most larger molecules out of the brain.

Tumors occurring inside the skull (intracranial) are named after the type of cell from which they developed. Examples are astrocytomas (from astrocytes), glioblastomas (from neuroglia cells), and melanomas (from melanocytes).

Tumors of the central nervous system are the most common type of solid tumor in children. In adults many intracranial malignacies are cancers that have spread from a distant site (secondary tumors from metastasis).

Summary

Like a union, each tissue is composed of one type of cell. It has its own size and character. And like a union, each tissue has a specific area of expertise. Epithelial tissue covers, lines, secretes, and absorbs. Connective tissue supports, connects, and protects from foreign invaders. Muscle tissue specializes in producing movement. Nervous tissue specializes in communication.

3

Organs and Organ Systems

*A*s cancer progresses from one cell into a tumor, it changes the organ's ability to function and disrupts the entire system to which the organ belongs. This chapter will help you understand the basic anatomy of the body and the organization of your organs. We have also included the types of cancers most common in the various organ systems.

Each of your cell citizens lives in a town. Some of the towns, such as the brain, heart, liver, and skin, are very large and perform an indispensable service. The great city of your heart, for example, is where large numbers of the muscle family live and work. These cells enjoy the harried existence of life in an essential organ. Other cells fancy the simple life of the heart suburbs, in the arteries and veins of the limbs. They prefer the reduced-stress lifestyle of a nonessential organ. Each organ-town is a composite of several different types of tissues. And even though the cells look different and come from different tissues, they all work together toward a common goal.

Each town and city also belongs to a larger organization with the same mission. Organ systems are composed of varying numbers and types of organs. They act together to perform a necessary job for the body. Each organ in the organ system depends upon the others, and each organ system is closely related to the other organ systems. For example, in the musculoskeletal system the skeleton is responsible for allowing the body to move. But it cannot provide the movement itself; for that function it must rely on the muscles. Working together, they get the body from here to there. The musculoskeletal system also works with other organ systems.

Within the bony safe of the long bones and pelvis lies the yellow bone marrow of the immune system and the red bone marrow of the blood system.

There are ten major organ systems: the integumentary system, skeletal system, muscular system, circulatory system, respiratory system, digestive system, nervous system, endocrine system, reproductive system, and urinary system. The immune system is different from the organ systems because it is made up of individual cells rather than organs. We will examine it separately.

The Integumentary System

The "integument" is another name for the skin, and the **integumentary system** includes the skin and its various attachments, including hair, finger- and toenails, lips, and skin glands. It is made up of a surface epithelial tissue lying atop a base of connective tissue.

In a general way, the skin's job is to keep the inside in and the outside out. The skin cells keep you watertight. Your skin prevents your bathwater from swelling you up like a sponge and your sunlamp from shriveling you into a raisin. The skin protects your insides from the environment. Your skin cell citizens prevent the illegal immigration of the vast majority of bacteria and viruses and block the entry of toxic chemicals.

The skin has other functions as well. It regulates body temperature through sweat, manufactures important chemicals such as vitamin D, and acts as a sensory organ for heat, cold, touch, pressure, and pain. The skin also excretes substances through your glands and pores. These substances include salts of various types and water.

Because the skin is exposed to many environmental factors, it is the most common site on the human body to form cancer. The most common forms of skin cancer are basal and squamous cell cancers caused by exposure to ultraviolet light. Melanoma, the more serious type of skin cancer, develops from melanocytes, the pigment-producing cells.

The Skeletal System

The skull, spine, rib cage, arm and leg bones, ligaments, tendons, and joints are included in the **skeletal system**. It is

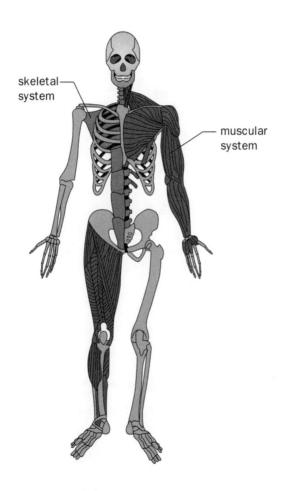

skeletal system

muscular system

Skeletal and muscular systems

almost entirely composed of two types of connective tissue: bone and cartilage. This system performs three major jobs:

1. The joints, or articulations, in the skeleton give the body the ability to move.
2. The bone tissue serves as a bank. Minerals such as calcium, magnesium, and phosphate can be deposited in the matrix and withdrawn when needed.
3. Hidden away in the safe-deposit box inside the bone is the red bone marrow. This tissue, a part of the blood system, is where red blood cells are made in the vital process called hemopoiesis.

Sarcomas of the bone tissue are rare and usually affect young persons. Most other cancers do not begin in the bone but have traveled (metastasized) there from other organs.

Muscular System

Muscle tissue can be organized into separate muscles that are considered individual organs. Together, they form the **muscular system**. The cells in a muscle have two major duties: movement and heat production. Although the joints of the skeletal system allow movement, they cannot make the movement themselves. For this they require the contraction of striated muscle. Movement inside the body cavity is provided by muscles made up of smooth muscle cells. For example, the movement of food through the digestive tract is provided by the smooth muscles in the esophagus, stomach, and intestines. Urine is moved through the urinary system by smooth muscles in the ureters, bladder, and urethra. Air is moved in and out of the lungs by smooth muscle in the diaphragm. The muscular system also serves as the major heat generator for the body, keeping tissues warm.

Muscle is made almost entirely of protein. When protein intake through food is low or when food protein is not digested or absorbed properly, it must come from some other source. That source is the muscle tissue. Even when enough protein is provided by the diet, cancer cells will raid the muscles for protein to change into glucose. When muscle tissue decreases, the individual muscle is less able to perform its job, causing weakness in movement and the sensation of coldness due to loss of heat production. Although cancer of the muscular system is very rare, cancer in general can cause a serious loss of muscle tissue.

Nervous System

The brain, spinal cord, and nerves are the organs of the **nervous system**. This system consists primarily of nervous tissue supported and protected by connective tissue.

The cell citizens of your nervous system work in several critical jobs. They are responsible for *rapid* cell-to-cell and organ-to-organ communication. Cells in these organs produce **neurotransmitters**, which initiate and sustain electric impulses. This allows your brain to talk to organs far and near, controlling, coordinating, and integrating their work.

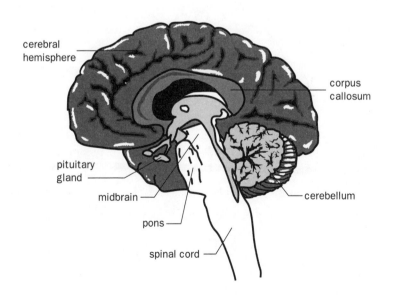

The brain

These messages travel very fast and provide only brief control. Nervous system cells also function as sensors. They are able to recognize heat, light, pressure, and temperature.

Cancers of the nervous system can be found in the gray matter of the brain, on the membrane covering the brain, and in the spinal cord. Endocrine glands located in the brain may also be a source of tumors. The skull is a common site for secondary tumors that have migrated from their place of origin.

Endocrine System

The **endocrine system** includes the pituitary and pineal glands; the hypothalamus, thyroid, and adrenal glands; the pancreas; and the testes or ovaries and placenta. These glands

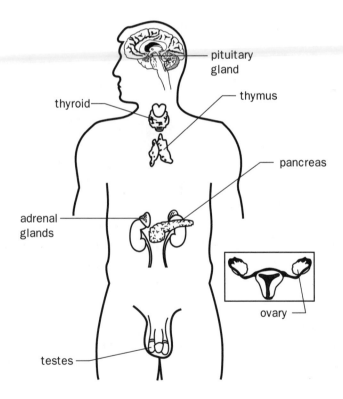

Endocrine system

release their hormones into the bloodstream directly, as opposed to the **exocrine glands**, which release their products into ducts.

The cell citizens of an endocrine gland are writers. They compose messages called **hormones**, which are distributed primarily through the bloodstream. Glands perform the same job as the nervous system: communication, integration, and control of bodily functions. The signals travel slower but are much longer lasting. Hormones are the main regulators of metabolism, growth and development, and reproduction.

Endocrine cell tumors are called **carcinoids**. Cancers of the endocrine system include the following:

- Germ cell cancers—These include testicular cancer (male), gestational trophoblasic neoplasms (placental), and ovarian cancer (female).
- Pancreatic cancer—Over 90 percent of the carcinomas of the pancreas are **mucinous adenocarcinomas** that originate in the pancreatic duct.
- Thyroid cancer.

Because they stimulate abnormal hormone production, cancers of the endocrine system are often able to produce symptoms in distant sites.

Circulatory System

Each cell citizen is connected to its fellow cells by means of a vast and intricate transport system of highways, roads, and lanes. We call this transportation network the **circulatory system**. It is composed of two parts: the cardiovascular system and the lymphatic system.

Cardiovascular System

The cardiovascular system has three main components: a liquid tissue called blood, a closed circuit of tubes through which the blood flows, and a pump to propel the blood.

Blood is the familiar salty red liquid that serves as the carrier in the cardiovascular system. The liquid part of blood, plasma, contains a vast and varied number of dissolved substances including vitamins, minerals, and other nutrients, blood sugar (glucose), insulin and other hormones used for communication, salts, enzymes, waste products from cells, and gases.

Suspended in the plasma is the solid portion of blood. It consists of the hemoglobin-containing red blood cells responsible for oxygen transport, the white blood cells of the immune system, and the platelets involved in blood-clot formation.

Blood travels through a series of tunnels called the blood vessels. The **arteries** carry oxygen-rich blood away from the heart to the tissues. The **veins** carry oxygen-depleted blood away from the tissues back to the heart. It is in the **capillaries**, the smallest blood vessels, where hungry tissues exchange carbon dioxide waste for oxygen. The oxygen-poor blood then drains into the veins.

The heart is at once the beginning and the end of the cardiovascular system. Made almost entirely of muscle, it functions as a four-chambered pump propelling oxygen-depleted blood from the tissues into the lungs. There the carbon dioxide from the tissues is exchanged for oxygen and the blood returns to the heart, which then pumps it out through the arteries.

Lymphatic System

The **lymphatic system** is made up of the lymphatic vessels, lymph nodes, lymph, thymus, and spleen. It transports fluids, large molecules, fat, and fat-related nutrients; it is also involved in the workings of the immune system. Major parts of the system include the lymph nodes, tonsils, thymus, spleen, and lymphatic vessels. Patches of lymphatic tissue are also found in isolated areas in the gastrointestinal tract, lungs, and bone marrow. The system also provides a means of return-

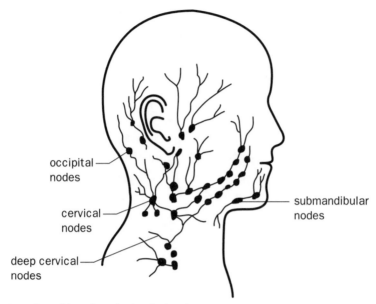

Location of lymph nodes in the head

ing liquid that escapes from the blood into the body tissues.

The lymph nodes are a combination police station and barracks. Round or kidney-shaped, these structures are usually found in groups around the body. You have between 500 and 1,500 lymph nodes that range in size from very tiny to about one inch in diameter. When nodes in the neck, armpits, or groin are enlarged, they can be felt. This is why your doctor pokes around your neck and abdomen.

The lymph system is used by the cells of the immune system. When an attacker such as a bacteria, virus, or cancer cell is picked up by one of the white blood cells, it is brought to the lymph node to be imprisoned and studied. When large numbers of these troublemakers are incarcerated, or when the immune army beefs up its security due to a threat, the bulging barracks can be felt by the doctor. Sometimes these nodes are removed during surgery. They are examined under a microscope to see if any cancer cells are present in the "jail." If the node has no cancer cells inside, your doctor knows that

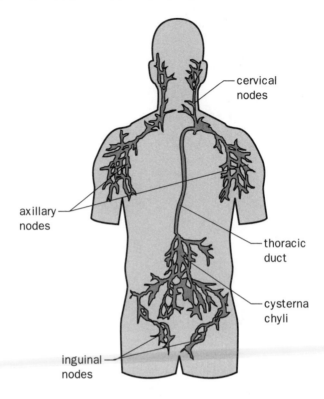

Lymphatic system

the cancer has not reached as far as the area drained by those nodes.

The organs involved in blood cell formation are a common site for cancer development. These types of cancer are called **leukemias**. Cancers of the lymph system are called **lymphomas**. The table in the preceding chapter listed common lymphatic cancers.

Respiratory System

The cells in your **respiratory system** are responsible for the exchange of carbon dioxide and oxygen between the air and the blood. Its organs include the nose, pharynx (throat), larynx, trachea, bronchi, and lungs.

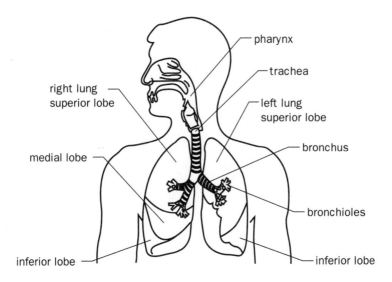

Respiratory system

Respiration involves two parallel processes. During external respiration (lung breathing), oxygen-rich air is brought into the lungs when you inhale, and carbon dioxide is removed from the body when you exhale. Through internal respiration (tissue breathing), oxygen in the red blood cells is exchanged for the waste carbon dioxide in the tissues.

When you inhale, the air is filtered and warmed by the nasal cavity and pharynx, then passes over the larynx on its way to the trachea. The trachea is composed of smooth muscle embedded with C-shaped cartilage rings, which function to keep the airway open at all times. As the trachea enters the chest, it divides into two branches called the **bronchi**, one of which leads to the right lung and the other to the left lung. Each of the bronchi divides into **bronchioles**, which end in the **alveoli**, or air sacs. Each alveolus resembles a small balloon that expands and contracts with the inhalation and exhalation of air. Beneath the thin membranes of the alveoli lie the capillary beds where the oxygen is collected by the red blood cells. Blood leaving the lungs is pulled into the heart and then pumped out through the arteries to oxygen-needy tissues.

Your two lungs are divided into lobes. The right lung has three lobes: upper, middle, and lower. The left lung has only two lobes: upper and lower. Between the lungs is the **mediastinum**, a cavity that contains the heart, aorta, esophagus, trachea, and bronchi. Each lung is covered by two membranes: the outer layer (called the parietal pleura) and the inner layer that lies on top of the lung (called the visceral pleura). The chest cavity is divided from the abdominal cavity by a muscular partition called the **diaphragm**. By contracting and relaxing, the diaphragm provides the pressure needed for respiration.

Each day your respiratory organs are exposed to over 10,000 liters of air containing toxins, dust, microorganisms, and other hazardous airborne particles. This makes those organs common sites for cancer. Carcinomas of the lung can be divided into four types:

1. Squamous cell carcinoma (30 to 35 percent of cases)
2. Adenocarcinoma (35 to 40 percent of cases)
3. Large-cell carcinoma (about 10 percent of cases)
4. Small-cell carcinoma (about 20 to 25 percent of cases)

These types are commonly grouped as small-cell carcinomas and non-small-cell carcinomas.

The Digestive System

The **digestive system** consists of the mouth, pharynx (throat), esophagus, stomach, intestines, rectum, and anus. These organs form a long, open-ended tube called the **alimentary canal** or the **gastrointestinal (GI) tract**. Accessory organs include the teeth, tongue, salivary glands, liver, gallbladder, and pancreas. The digestive tract digests food, absorbs nutrients, and eliminates feces (bodily waste). The entire alimentary canal is lined with epithelial cells. When

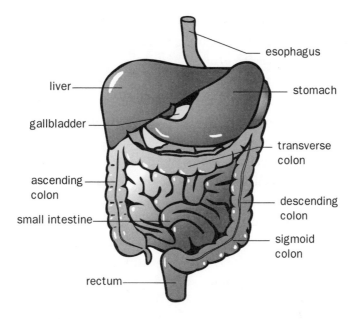

Digestive System

the replacement of these fast-growing cells is halted as a result of chemotherapy or radiation, painful side effects such as mouth sores, sore throat, and stomach upset can result. Damage to the epithelium of the small intestine, however, causes more than just discomfort. It can result in electrolyte loss through diarrhea or malnutrition from malabsorption.

The main function of the epithelium of the small intestine is to absorb nutrients. This is reflected in its unusual structure. The lining of the small intestine is wrinkled with velvety folds called rugae. The rugae are covered with millions of small fingerlike projections called villi. Each villus is one millimeter in height and has a small artery, a vein, and lymph vessel running through its center. It is covered with a single layer of cells that have even finer projections on their top exposed surfaces called microvilli. Each cell on the villus has about 1,700 of them. Under the microscope, the microvilli projecting out from the end of each villus give the appearance of a paintbrush and are referred to as the "brush bor-der." Enzymes necessary to digest foods are produced in the brush border near the top of each villi. The digested nutri-ents then pass through the villi walls into the blood or lymph vessels. This arrangement of villi and microvilli increases the absorptive area of the small intestine to about 250 square meters, the size of a small tennis court.

When cancer treatments such as radiation or chemother-apy injure the cells of the villi, some nutrients can no longer be digested (due to the loss of the enzymes) or absorbed (due to the loss of the microvilli and villi). This can result in malnutrition.

Since the digestive system is open to the environment and its toxins, it is a common site for cancer development. We will divide it into three parts: the mouth, esophagus, and stomach; the accessory organs of the liver and biliary tract; and the small and large intestines.

Cancers of the Upper Aerodigestive Tract

The upper aerodigestive tract includes the structures you use to eat and breathe, including the lips, mouth, tongue, nose, nasal sinuses, throat, salivary glands, and neck. Squamous cell carcinoma is by far the most common type of cancer to occur in this area. This type of cancer is strongly related to expo-sure to environmental toxins such as alcohol, tobacco leaves or smoke, and industrial chemicals. Since all of the surfaces in touch with the toxins are at risk, once a cancer develops on one structure, it is not uncommon to find independent lesions on other nearby surfaces. To prevent the disease from recurring and to allow the epithelial tissues to become healthy again, you must stop the exposure to the toxins.

Sometimes surgery to remove cancerous lesions can result in eating difficulties. When this occurs, it is important that you see a certified nutritionist or dietitian to help you get the nourishment your body needs to heal itself.

Cancers of the Esophagus, Stomach, and Small Intestine

Half of esophageal cancers occur in the middle third of the organ, with the remainder evenly divided between the upper and lower thirds. Most cancers of the first two segments are squamous cell carcinomas. Those in the lower third are usually adenocarcinomas. Gastric cancers (*gastric* means "of the stomach") are usually adenocarcinomas. Cancers of the small intestine are very rare. They are usually carcinoids, developed from the endocrine cells scattered throughout the small intestine, or lymphomas, developed from the lymphoid cells in the intestine.

Colorectal Cancers

Malignancies of the colon, rectum, and anus are classified as colorectal cancers. The colon is the most common site for tumors in the gastrointestinal tract. The American Cancer Society estimates that there are approximately 151,000 new cases of colorectal cancer each year in the United States. Ninety-eight percent of colorectal cancers are carcinomas, with 60 to 70 percent occurring in the lower third of the colon and rectum.

Liver and Biliary Tract Cancers

The liver is the largest glandular organ of your body overseeing and managing the internal environment. It has a wide variety of jobs:

- It receives, via the portal vein, all of the nutrient-rich blood from the intestines and is involved in fat, protein, and carbohydrate metabolism.
- It is responsible for detoxifying (making harmless) a wide variety of substances.
- It serves as a storehouse for excess vitamins B_{12}, A, and D and the mineral iron.
- It is an exocrine gland, producing about a pint of bile each

day. Bile works as an emulsifier, allowing fats and fat-soluble nutrients to dissolve in the watery lymph. Without an adequate supply of bile, fat is not absorbed properly (a condition called **steatorrhea**).

Because its job is so important, the liver has a tremendous ability to regenerate. If large areas of cells are killed or removed but the remaining section is healthy, the liver will regrow and resume most of its functions.

The **biliary system** includes the gallbladder, which stores the bile made in the liver, and the ducts of the liver, gallbladder, and pancreas. The right and left **extrahepatic ducts** exit the liver and then join to form the **common hepatic duct**. These ducts carry bile. The **cystic duct** from the gallbladder joins the common hepatic duct to form the **common bile duct**. Bile can either leave the gallbladder through the cystic duct on its way to the duodenum or enter the gallbladder, where it is stored until needed. The common bile duct is joined by the pancreatic duct carrying digestive enzymes just before entering the duodenum at the peri-ampulla of Vater.

The most commonly occurring cancer of the liver is **hepatocellular carcinoma**. However, most hepatic (liver) cancers are metastases from primary tumors of the breast, lung, and gastrointestinal tract. Biliary tract cancers include carcinomas of the gallbladder, the extrahepatic biliary ducts, and the peri-ampulla of Vater.

Urinary System

The job of cleaning up the bloodstream falls to the cells of the urinary system, which includes a pair of kidneys and ureters, the bladder, and the urethra. Together, the fist-sized kidneys filter over 1,700 liters of blood each day to produce about 1 liter of highly concentrated urine. Urine can be compared to used wash water. It contains the waste products that have been dumped into the bloodstream by other organs.

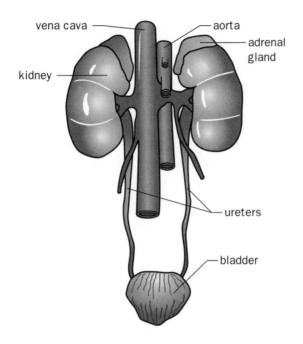

vena cava

aorta

adrenal gland

kidney

ureters

bladder

Urinary system

Urine drips from the kidney down through a long tube called the ureter until it reaches the bladder. The bladder is a hollow muscular organ that expands as it fills with urine. Urine is temporarily stored here, exiting through the urethra during micturition (urination). The kidneys also aid in maintaining the balance of electrolytes, water, and acid. The most common cancers of the kidneys are renal cell carcinoma (also called hypernephroma or adenocarcinoma of the kidney), which accounts for 85 to 90 percent of all renal (kidney) cancers; Wilms' tumor (also called nephroblastoma), which is a childhood tumor; and urothelial carcinomas of the renal pelvis. Cancers of the ureters are rare and are usually secondary tumors from metastasis. The most common forms of bladder cancer are transitional cell carcinoma, which accounts for 90 percent of bladder carcinomas; squamous cell carcinoma; and mixed transitional and squamous cell carcinoma. Adenomas of the bladder are rare and include signet cell carcinoma and mesonephric or nephrogenic adenoma. Secondary tumors can also occur from cancers in the cervix, uterus, prostate, and rectum. Most cancers of the urethra are squamous cell cancers.

Male Reproductive System

The **male reproductive system** includes: the male gonads or testes, where sperm is manufactured; genital ducts (epididymis, vas deferens, ejaculatory ducts, and urethra); and the supporting structures (scrotum, penis, and spermatic cords). The cells of the male reproductive system are dedicated to the manufacture, transport, and introduction of sperm into the female tract.

Testes and Epididymis

The **testes** are a pair of organs located in an external sac called the **scrotum**. They are both a production site for sperm and a gland that secretes the male hormone, testos-

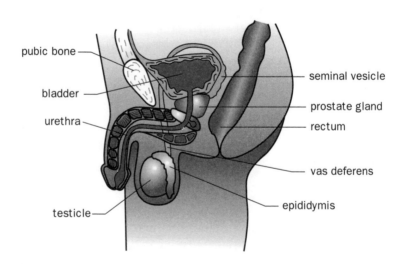

Male reproductive system

terone. Sperm created in the testes exit through the **epididymis**, a very long but thin, tightly coiled tube. Here the sperm are allowed to mature for one to three weeks before passing through the ejaculatory duct in the penis. The genital ducts are surrounded by a layer of tough connective tissue.

Over 95 percent of testicular malignancies are germ cell cancers. Germ cell cancer can be divided into two major types: **seminomas** and **nonseminomatous germ cell tumors**, including embryonal carcinomas, yolk sac tumors, choriocarcinomas, teratomas, and tumors that are a combination of these types.

Prostate

The **prostate** is a doughnut-shaped gland that surrounds the urethra. It produces a thin alkaline substance that forms the largest part of the seminal fluid. Carcinoma of the prostate is the most common form of cancer in men. Over 100,000 new cases are detected each year.

Penis

The two types of penile cancer are carcinoma of the penis and carcinoma in situ, a type of carcinoma where the malignant cells have not penetrated into the adjacent tissues or metastasized to distant sites.

Female Reproductive System

The **female reproductive system** includes the female gonads (ovaries), the genital ducts (uterus, fallopian tubes, and vagina), and the supporting structures (**mammary glands**, or breasts, and **vulva** or genitalia). The female tract manufactures the **ova** (egg), accepts sperm, fosters fertilization, and allows development, birth, and nourishment of the offspring.

Breast cancer is the most common malignancy in women

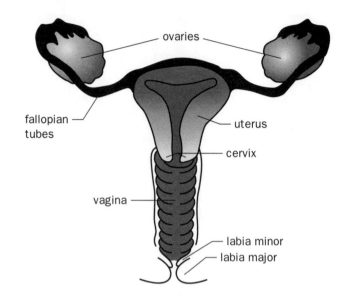

Female reproductive system

of the western world. According to the American Cancer Society, approximately 143,000 new cases are diagnosed each year. Cancers of the breast include infiltrating ductal carcinoma, infiltrating lobular carcinoma, cystosarcoma phylloides, and intraductal carcinoma (ductal carcinoma in situ, or DCIS).

Malignancies associated with the genital tract include invasive squamous cell carcinomas of the cervix, vulva, and vagina; clear cell adenocarcinomas of the vagina; endometrial carcinoma; and choriocarcinoma.

Cancers of the ovary include the epithelial carcinomas (serous, endometroid, clear cell, and mucinous); the malignant germ cell tumors (dysgerminoma, yolk sac tumor, and immature teratoma); and sex cord stromal (granulosa cell) tumors.

The growth of healthy reproductive tissue is regulated by the sex hormones. Cancers arising from these tissues will also respond to hormones by increasing the rate at which they grow.

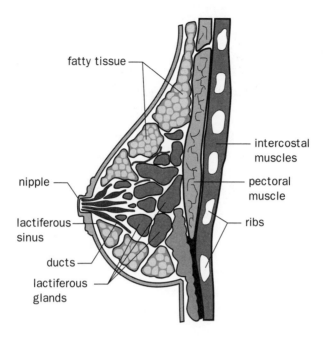

Side view of breast

Summary

Tissues are organized into organs that perform a specific function. This is much like a city where several unions (tissues) supply workers dedicated to a common function. The organs of the body are further organized into organ systems or industries: groups of cities and towns that produce similar products or services. There are ten major organ systems in the human body. What affects one organ will affect the entire organ system and thus the ability of that system to do its part in production and tissue maintainance.

4

Cancer:
When Good Cells Go Bad

*A*n understanding of cancer growth and tumors requires knowledge of how a normal cell is transformed into a malignant cell. This chapter will follow the life a single cancer cell from the beginning to its transformation to its spread to other organs. It is important to understand the stages of cancer development because they hold the key to treatment.

Occasionally, a cell becomes discontented with the status quo. A disgruntled worker, it does not want anyone to tell it how to live, where to live, or how to reproduce. It loses its ability to grow and differentiate normally. This insurgent can clone copies of itself until there is a whole clan pursuing the dubious goal of anarchy. As the numbers increase, some of the anarchists hop into the bloodstream transport system and travel to other organ cities, where they cause further disruption. They infiltrate the tissue unions and cause strikes. If left unchecked, these dissidents can ultimately interrupt food supply and totally disrupt the order of the body.

In a city with billions of residents, dissidents are not uncommon. The immune police force has many techniques for finding and arresting these troublemakers.

Carcinogenesis is the process by which a normal cell citizen is converted into a cancer anarchist. This force is thought to take the form of a mutation—a change to the genetic material in the nucleus of the cell. Such changes can be in the phosphate groups, the order of the bases, or in the three-dimensional structure of the DNA molecule. Many types of substances can cause mutations; environmental toxins, viruses, and radiation are some of the most common.

Mutation is a common event in the life of a cell, with several thousand errors introduced into your DNA each and every day. Cell citizens are bombarded every day with a wide variety of carcinogens. Some occur naturally, such as aflatoxin from the mold *Aspergillus flavus* and nitrosamines produced in the gastrointestinal tract. Others fall on us from the sky like the sun's ultraviolet rays or seep up at us from below like radon present in soil and rock gas. Numerous human-made chemicals are inhaled as cigarette smoke or industrial pollution. Asbestos fibers, polychlorinated biphenyls (PCBs), some insecticides, and vinyl chloride are other manufactured carcinogens.

Very often a mutation can be corrected by special enzymes that patrol the molecule, looking for mistakes. Over twenty different enzymes are dedicated to "spell-checking" your DNA words. Substances found in foods can increase the ability of these enzymes to seek and fix mutations. Also, many mutations occur in a genetic sequence that is crucial for survival, causing the cell to die before passing on the mutation. Only cells that survive these protective mechanisms have the potential to become cancerous.

Unfortunately, in spite of these defenses, carcinogenesis occasionally takes place. The process consists of three stages: initiation, promotion, and progression. Nutrition has an impact on all three.

Carcinogenesis: The Beginning of Cancer

A cell does not decide on its own to become an anarchist. It must first be **initiated**. If the mutation is not fixed and the cell divides and produces a copy of itself with the same mutation, then initiation is said to have occurred. Once initiation is completed, it cannot be undone.

The initiated cell is not a tumor cell. It can become a tumor cell only if it is acted upon by a **promoter**. In the majority of cases, this does not happen, and the cancerous cell dies without having spread its seditious manifesto. Promoters are substances that promote tumor growth in initiated cells. They have no effect on normal cells. Researchers believe that promoters do not work by changing the structure of DNA, since the effects of promotion are not permanent and can be reversed. The initiated cell must be constantly exposed to the promoter for tumor growth to occur. Promoters also alter the ability of cells to differentiate, producing cells that cannot mature. Some carcinogens are both initiators and promoters. They are called complete carcinogens. The female hormone estrogen is a cancer promoter in hormone-dependent cancers.

As the promoted cells multiply, they are very susceptible to another class of compounds called **progressive agents**. Progressive agents cause the promoted cells to reproduce. These agents cause further damage to the chromosomes, resulting in a cell that loses the ability to look and act like its surrounding neighbors. Progression, like initiation, cannot be reversed.

Cancerous Tumors

Cancer comes from the Latin word for crab. Like a crab, cancer attaches itself to tissues and organs and hangs on obstinately. We often speak of cancer as if it were one specific disease, but this is not the case. Cancer is a group of diseases that share a common characteristic: cells that divide at a much greater rate than normal, causing masses of tissue called tumors. **Oncology** (*oncos* means tumor in Greek) is the study of **neoplasia** (*neo* = new, *plasia* = growth). A new growth is then called a **neoplasm**, another word for tumor.

A tumor acts as a parasite, competing with normal tissues for food and energy. There are two types of tumors: benign and malignant. **Benign tumors** grow slowly and stay in one place. **Malignant**, or cancerous, **tumors** usually grow rapidly and can spread to distant tissues by a process called **metastasis**. Some of the malignant cells detach from the tumor and travel to other parts of the body, usually through the blood or lymph vessels.

Malignant tumors are classified as either carcinomas or sarcomas. Carcinomas develop from epithelial and endothelial tissue such as the breast, skin, and lung and metastasize primarily to nearby tissues through the lymph system. Sar-

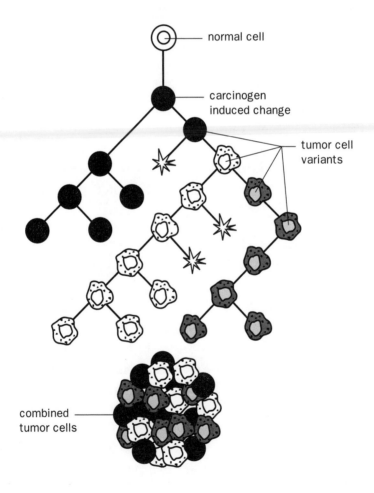

normal cell

carcinogen induced change

tumor cell variants

combined tumor cells

comas arise from mesoderm tissue such as muscle, cartilage, and bone and spread primarily through the bloodstream. A tumor's histologic type is determined by the appearance and organization of the cells under a microscope.

All tumors have two basic parts:

1. The **parenchyma**, which is made up of the dividing and growing neoplastic cells. These cells determine the nature and type of the growth.

2. The **stroma**, which is the supportive tissue made up of connective tissue and blood vessels. Without stromal support, a tumor would not survive. The stromal blood supply keeps the tumor supplied with food, and connective tissue provides a framework for the parenchyma.

Cancer treatments can target the parenchymal tissues, the stromal tissues, or both. Nutrition therapy also can affect both types of cancer tissues.

Tumors

Most malignant tumors have grown from a single transformed cell. These clone cells are extremely susceptible to further mutation, producing strains of subclones. Subclones that lie low and do not call attention to themselves will not attract the interest of the immune system. These cells live longer and are able to multiply. Subclones that do provoke the immune system are promptly killed by white blood cells. Subclones that have high needs for nutrients will not grow or spread as fast as those that thrive in a low-oxygen, low-energy environment. Like all life forms, the strongest survive.

Cells in cancerous tumors exhibit some important differences from their normal counterparts:

- Since the malignant cells are anarchists at heart, they grow in disorderly masses, uninhibited by contact with other cells. And unlike normal cells, which like to be "tied" to a solid surface, malignant cells will flourish while floating free.

- Malignant cells never mature. They never differentiate into specialized cells. They are stuck in a sort of permanent adolescence, keeping their ability to reproduce but never differentiating into a particular type of cell with a normal job.
- Malignant cells are immortal. Normal cells differentiate and eventually die after a number of divisions. Some malignant cells have grown in culture dishes for decades.

Cancer tumors are able to grow by infiltration, invasion, and destruction of the surrounding tissue.

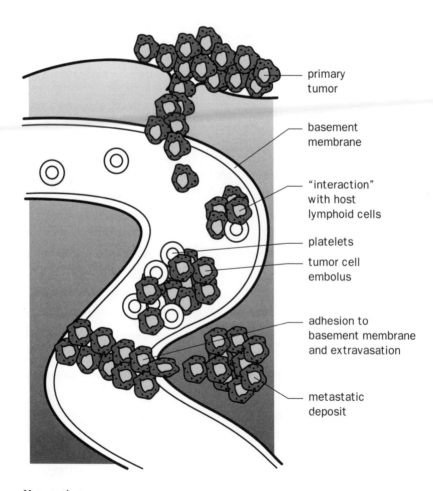

primary
tumor

basement
membrane

"interaction"
with host
lymphoid cells

platelets

tumor cell
embolus

adhesion to
basement membrane
and extravasation

metastatic
deposit

Metastatic tumor

Invasion

For a clone cell from a tumor to spread, it must (1) find a way to get out of the surrounding normal tissue, (2) push its way through the blood vessel wall, and (3) be able to reverse the process to set up housekeeping at a distant site. This process is illustrated on the previous page. The connective tissue that surrounds the tumor and basement membrane of blood vessel walls is called the **extracellular matrix**. Cancer cells can secrete enzymes that dissolve the extracellular matrix, forming a tunnel for the cells to travel through. Some of the compounds that are formed from this breakdown are growth promoting.

Once the cell is circulating in the blood, it is very susceptible to the immune system army, particularly the "natural killer" (NK) cells, described in the next chapter. Metastasis can be slowed by keeping your NK cells fed and healthy.

Staging Tumors

To describe the extent of the disease at the time of diagnosis, oncologists describe the tumor with a system of **staging**. Using this system helps your oncologist plan your treatment and compare different treatment approaches. The most frequently used system of staging is the TNM **classification** proposed by the American Joint Commission on Cancer:

- The *T* (for tumor) stands for the primary tumor or the place the cancer originated. The higher the number next to the *T*, the larger the tumor and the greater its involvement with surrounding tissues. The lowest number, T0, represents cancer that has not invaded the local tissues. This is also called cancer "in situ." The highest number, T4, represents a very large tumor that has penetrated the local tissues and grown into other organs.
- The *N* (for nodes) stands for the local or regional lymph nodes that drain the area of the primary tumor. The extent of node involvement goes from N0 for no node involvement to N4 for extensive involvement.

- The *M* (for metastasis) denotes the absence (M0) or presence (M1) of metastasis, or spread.

Therefore, a TCM assignment of T0 N0 M0 indicates a cancer that has not invaded the local tissues (cancer in situ) and that has no lymph node involvement and no metastasis. A T3 N3 M1 assignment indicates a cancer with a large tumor that has grown extensively into the local tissue, a great deal of lymph node involvement, and metastasis.

The TCM assignments are grouped into four stages, expressed as Roman numerals I through IV. Stage I cancers are small and localized, while stage IV cancers are metastic. How the TCM assignments are staged differs from tumor to tumor.

Summary

Carcinogenesis involves multiple stages, multiple genes, and probably multiple mechanisms. Tumors arise when cell growth is not properly regulated by the genes. One way this can happen is when mutations occur. Mutations are changes in the cell's DNA. Even small changes in the DNA can cause big problems for the individual cell, tissue, or entire body. Certain chemicals and types of radiation can cause changes in the genes or chromosomes. Mutations may involve the number of chromosomes, or a gain or loss or rearrangement of chromosome segments. Because mutations can be deadly, the body has a number of ways to prevent or fix the damage.

5

....

The Body Fights Back

*M*utations are a common event in the life of a cell, and the body has developed mechanisms to prevent these mutations from doing damage. This chapter will introduce you to two of these mechanisms: the immune system and the antioxidant system. The immune system elements patrol the circulatory system and organs of the body on an antigen seek-and-destroy mission. The anti-oxidant system uses a group of substances to protect cells and tissues. This chapter will look at how these defense systems fight to free your body of cancer. It also identifies foods and nutrients necessary to support these systems.

When we think of the war on crime, we imagine police chasing robbers, muggers, and drug pushers. Often their efforts are not enough, and crime becomes an unavoidable complication of community life. But there is a place where such a war is fought and won on a daily basis—your body. In the microscopic world, the human body is surrounded by toxic gases, free radicals, damaging radiation, bacteria, viruses, parasites, and other sources of harm. The human body has two mechanisms for dealing with these situations: the immune system, which prevents the invasion of organisms, and the antioxidant system, which prevents damage from oxidation.

Recently science has recognized the critical role these systems play in cancer prevention. Often overlooked, however, are their ability to destroy cancers already present and the overwhelming importance of adequate nutrition to keep these systems running at peak efficiency.

The Immune System

The human body is gifted with the ability to keep itself free from disease-causing invaders. This immunity (from the Latin *immunitas,* meaning "freedom from disease") is achieved by the **immune system**. The immune system is at once the smallest and the largest body system. Unlike the organ systems described in the previous chapter, the immune system has no major organs of its own. It is composed of individual microscopic cells and molecules that have widespread access to every nook and cranny of the body. These cells include lymphocytes (white blood cells), phagocytes, and natural killer cells, and these molecules include antibodies, complement, and interferon.

These immune elements see approaching objects in terms of black and white, as either bad or good. Scientists do not yet know how they do this and what criteria they use for classification. One theory is that the immune system somehow can tell the difference between the cell citizens, tissues, and proteins that belong to their body ("self") and all other proteins ("nonself"). A more recent theory suggests that the immune system discerns the difference between anything that causes cell stress or lytic cell death (the dangerous) and that which does not cause cell stress or death. It does this by listening for "danger signals."

The Antigen-Antibody Response

The nonself or dangerous proteins are called **antigens**. Antigens may be peptides embedded in a living cell wall, fragments from a destroyed foreign cell, or stray proteins. A specific antigen stimulates the immune cells to manufacture a specific **antibody**. Antibodies, sometimes called immunoglobulins, are protein molecules that react only with their matching antigen, as a key fits into one specific lock. They can be located on the surface of a leukocyte as a receptor site or secreted as water-soluble antibodies that can travel far from the manufacturing cell. The antibody-antigen reaction sometimes renders the antigen harmless. Other times antibodies form a tasty coating on antigens, thereby attracting hungry scavenger cells.

Phagocytic Cells

The body's scavengers, called **phagocytes**, include **monocytes**, **neutrophils**, and other antigen-capturing white blood cells. They wander the highways and byways of the body, looking for something good to eat (phagocytize).

When a neutrophil finds a "nonself" cell or protein (or one that is broadcasting a danger signal), it simply eats it. The ingested particle is then killed with free radical bullets, described later in this chapter.

Monocytes patrol the blood. Some of them wander into the tissues where they transform into cells called **macrophages**. These cells are even more helpful to the immune soldiers than neutrophils. When a macrophage encounters an antigen, it swallows, digests, and displays the antigen as a fragment on its cell surface. The fragment serves as a sort of memento of what the macrophage has found in its travels, and it is used to make antibodies. Macrophages can also be summoned to infected areas by messages broadcast by lymphocytes, as described later in this chapter. These macrophages are more able to kill microorganisms.

Phagocytes are also the cleanup crew after an immune battle. They eat the bodies of the dead lymphocytes and bacteria so that the corpses do not contribute to an infection.

Lymphocytes

Lymphocytes (white blood cells) are the infantrymen of the immune army. They come in two different types: **T cells** (or T lymphocytes), which are born in the thymus gland, and **B cells**, which are born in the bone marrow. Each T or B cell is programmed to recognize only one specific antibody by means of antigen receptor sites embedded on the cellular membrane. Each type of antigen has a corresponding B and T cell.

T lymphocytes are in charge of the cellular immunity division of the infantry. They are divided into two major types: the **helper-inducer T cells** and the **cytotoxic-suppresser killer T cells**. Helper T cells must be present to help B cells produce antibody. Cytotoxic are regulatory cells.

The cytotoxic T cells are the most aggressive fighters in the army. They are able to detect spies: cells that appear normal on the outside but harbor a virus or mutated genes on the inside. Acting as both judge and executioner, the cytotoxic T cell decides who is abnormal and then kills the defective cell by riddling its cellular membrane with holes or poisoning it with lethal toxins.

T cells cannot recognize antibodies circulating in the blood. They will react only to processed antibodies found by the macrophages and monocytes of the phagocytic system.

The B cells control the **humoral immunity** division of the infantry. They can manufacture enormous copies of the antibodies they display on their membranes. These water-soluble antibodies travel in the circulatory system, quickly seeking out their victims.

Natural Killer Cells

In the fight against cancer, the most important cell is the **natural killer (NK) cell**. Unlike killer T cells, NK cells do not need to be activated by an antigen. This means that they are able to attack and kill a wide variety of cells they have never seen before. After activation by a molecule called interleukin-2, NK cells can kill a wide variety of human tumor cells that are not even recognized by the T and B cells. Keeping these super soldiers in optimal fighting condition is therefore necessary to beat cancer.

The Immune Response

Once a protein fragment has been displayed on the surface of an antigen-displaying cell, a corresponding antibody then appears on both a B and a T cell. Then when a T cell with a specific antibody on its surface encounters an antigen-displaying cell with the corresponding antigen on its surface, it becomes activated. Activated T cells send an alarm to other lymphocytes that an intruder has been discovered. They do this by secreting chemical messengers called **lymphokines**.

These specific lymphokines alert the corresponding B cells that the intruder has again been found. Some B cells respond to the alert by transforming into rapidly dividing plasma cells. Plasma cells are mobile antibody factories. Each plasma cell manufactures a specific antibody at the rate of ten million antibody molecules per hour.

Lymph Tissue

All of the immune cells travel in the bloodstream until they reach one of many secondary organs of the lymph system, such as the lymph nodes, spleen, or tonsils. There they congregate and mix with others, communicating with lymphokines and trading information on the types of antigens they have encountered in their travels. As many as one billion white blood cells can be found in as little as one gram of lymph tissue. When an antigen activates T and B cells, greatly increasing cell division, the increasing population of the lymph nodes can be felt by a physician. Swollen lymph nodes are a sign that an antigen has been found.

Nutrition and the Immune System

Like all armies, the immune system marches on its stomach. The adult body produces 126 billion neutrophils every day. Normally about 25 billion are patrolling the blood, and another 2½ trillion are stationed in the bone marrow. Ten trillion lymphocytes are housed in the lymph tissues. This all adds up to a huge food bill. If these soldiers do not get the necessary nourishment, they will not be able to carry out their responsibilities or have energy for reproduction.

A lack of many trace minerals and vitamins will decrease the activity of these soldiers. The following list summarizes how some of these shortages affect the immune system:

- *Zinc*—A shortage causes a decrease in T killer cell and NK cell activity.
- *Iron*—A deficiency reduces NK cell cytotoxicity, phagocytosis, and killing capacity of neutrophils.
- *Copper*—A lack reduces the population of T cells and depresses the immune system.
- *Selenium*—A deficiency decreases antibody production.
- *Selenium and Vitamin E*—a shortage of these two synergistic nutrients will decrease the cytotoxic function of NK cells.
- *Pyridoxine*—A lack of this B vitamin reduces antibody production and decreases the ability of lymphocytes to function.

The following vitamins also affect the immune system:

- *Vitamin C*—An antioxidant nutrient that protects the watery areas of the cell from the "friendly fire" of cancer treatment. As an antihistamine, it detoxifies histamine, which can depress the immune system.
- *Vitamin E*—This antioxidant nutrient protects the lipid components of cells, including the cell membrane and the membranes surrounding various organelles. It works synergistically with selenium.
- *Vitamin A*—This fat-soluble vitamin inhibits the growth and development of cancer. A deficiency decreases the number of plasma cells producing antibody.

But strong warriors are only part of the story. The immune fighters must also be properly armed and able to transmit and receive communications. The molecules needed for this are formed from protein, and so a lack of this macronutrient will decrease the amount of antibody bombs the army can produce and reduce the number of messages exchanged.

Protective elements also are important. Antioxidant nutrients and phytochemicals are needed to enhance these systems and protect healthy cells from treatment-induced free radicals (a harmful type of molecule described in the next section).

Fats such as fish and flaxseed oil inhibit the ability of cancer cells to spread by hindering attachment. The types of dietary fatty acids influence the composition and fluidity of macrophage membranes, impairing their ability to kill tumor cells. When animals are fed diets high in polyunsaturated or saturated fats, the cytotoxic abilities of macrophages decrease.

Free Radicals

One of the most common causes of cellular injury and death is damage from free radicals. It can be caused by radiation and chemical injury, cellular aging, microbial killing by phagocytic cells, inflammatory damage, and tumor destruction by macrophages.

A **free radical** is a molecule that has a single unpaired electron in its outer orbit. Electrons have a compulsion to travel in pairs, and molecules that lack an electron will go to almost any length to acquire a new partner. They will react with lipids, proteins, or carbohydrates. Particularly vulnerable are the components of the cellular membrane and DNA. Once this reaction occurs, the molecule is no longer reactive. However, the molecule it got the electron from is now reactive and looking for another electron, starting a chain reaction of damage.

The body has two main mechanisms for ridding itself of free radicals:

1. It can obtain **antioxidants** (agents that protect against electron loss to free radicals) manufacturing them inside the body or obtaining them from the diet.
2. The body also has a system of enzymes to neutralize the free radicals generated as a result of normal metabolism.

Antioxidant Nutrients

The most commonly recognized antioxidant nutrients are beta-carotene (a precursor to vitamin A), vitamins C and E, and selenium. They are, however, but a tip of the iceberg. Beta-carotene is just one of many carotenoids with antioxidant properties, not the most powerful. Other powerful carotenes include alpha-carotene, lycopene, lutein, and cryptoxanthin.

Flavonoids, like carotenoids, are a large family of pigments. Those with antioxidant activity include rutin, quercetin, myricetin, and the citrus flavones. Other pigments that neutralize free radicals are the proanthocyanidins, tannins, and anthocyanins.

Antioxidant Enzymes

Enzymes needed by the human body are manufactured using DNA templates. Although certain vitamins, minerals, and phytochemicals (bioactive plant chemicals) act as free radical quenchers, the body's primary defense against free radicals is its enzyme systems. These systems produce the weapons with which the immune army attacks invaders and insurgents. The major enzymes used by the body are glutathione peroxidase, superoxide dismutase, and catalase.

Glutathione Peroxidase

Glutathione peroxidase is used primarily by the cells of the liver, lungs, heart, and blood to deactivate free radicals before they can cause injury. It inactivates the hydrogen peroxide free radical and scavenges lipid peroxides, the free radicals formed when oxygen radicals attack the unsaturated fatty acids of the cell membranes. As a result, the cell membrane loses two essential fatty acids: arachidonic acid and linoleic acid. This loss increases the permeability of the membrane, leading to an imbalance of minerals including calcium, magnesium, sodium, and potassium.

Selenium is a part or cofactor of this enzyme, and vitamins C and E enhance its effects. In fact, some studies suggest that combining selenium and vitamin E with glutathione is more effective for cancer prevention than using either alone. Glutathione and the amino acid cystine can increase levels of glutathione peroxidase. Glutathione is found in many foods, or it can be supplemented.

Superoxide Dismutase and Catalase

Cells use **superoxide dismutase (SOD)** to prevent damage by the superoxide free radical. If not quenched, the superoxide free radical degenerates into the lethal hydroxyl radical. SOD prevents this by demoting the superoxide radical to the less toxic hydrogen peroxide. The hydroxyl radical is dangerous because it can steal electrons from virtually any organic molecule in the immediate area.

When SOD works in the mitochondria, it requires manganese. When used in the cytoplasm, it requires copper and zinc.

Catalase is the enzyme that completes the reaction started by SOD. It does so by reducing the hydrogen peroxide radical to oxygen and water. Catalase performs its work in the blood and the peroxisomes (enzyme-containing organelles) of cells. It requires the mineral iron as a cofactor.

Summary

The immune system is like an army with a vast contingent of soldiers, including lymphocytes, phagocytes, macrophages, and natural killer (NK) cells. These cells either kill invaders directly or secrete substances that kill them indirectly. Proper nutrition is necessary to feed the immune cells and provide the antioxidants necessary to protect healthy cells from cancer treatment. Like all armies, the immune army must be well fed in order to fight. The nutrients it needs can sometimes be supplemented. But the supplementation in turn must be supplemented by healthy amounts of fruits, vegetables, whole grains, and other whole foods. This will ensure that you get all of the nutrients, known and unknown, that your immune army needs.

6

Carbohydrates and Cancer

Carbohydrates are made by plants as a way of storing energy from the sun. In the human diet, carbohydrates provide most of the energy for the cell citizens. They are carried in the blood as glucose and regulated by the hormone insulin. A high blood sugar level feeds cancer tumors. This chapter explores the effect of carbohydrates on blood sugar and cancer.

Without a doubt, my favorite macronutrient is the carbohydrate. It fills the stomach and calms the mind as no other nutrient can. There are three general types of carbohydrates: simple, digestible, and indigestible.

Monosaccharides

Simple carbohydrates, or sugars, are easily recognized in foods because of their sweet taste. The basic unit of the carbohydrate is the **monosaccharide** (*mono* = one, *saccharide* = sugar), and the main carbohydrate of the body is glucose (blood sugar). Other monosaccharides you may be familiar with are **fructose** (the main sugar in fruit) and **galactose** (the sugar that, together with glucose, forms lactose or milk sugar).

Monosaccharides are classified by how many carbon atoms they have. Fructose, glucose, and galactose all are made of six carbons in a ring. Actually these simple sugars are all composed of the same elements: six carbon, twelve oxygen, and twelve hydrogen atoms arranged in a ring. They are called **hexoses** (*hex* = six, *ose* = sugar). The molecular formula is written as: $C_6H_{12}O_6$.

The purpose of eating carbohydrates and most fats is to

provide the body with glucose. Glucose provides the fuel for almost all cells and is the only form in which sugar can be transported in the bloodstream. For example, your central nervous system uses nine tablespoons of glucose each day, and your red blood cells use three tablespoons.

Disaccharides

Two joined monosaccharides form a **disaccharide** (*di* = two). Three disaccharides are found in the food you eat. **Sucrose** is the disaccharide you are probably most familiar with, since it is the sole component of refined white sugar. It is made up of one molecule of glucose joined to one molecule of fructose. **Lactose** is found only in milk and enhances the absorption of its calcium. Lactose is composed of one glucose molecule and one galactose molecule. **Maltose** is composed of two glucose molecules. It is found only in germinating cereals and is used to make malt beverages. Barley malt syrup is a tasty alternative to refined sugar.

The enzymes **sucrase** and **lactase** are necessary to break apart sucrose and lactose into its component monosaccharides. These two sugars lie on top of the microvilli of the small intestine. Anything that injures the microvilli, such as radiation and chemotherapy, will affect the body's ability to digest and absorb these sugars. This results in the sucrose or lactose reaching the colon undigested, where it attracts water, resulting in diarrhea. In addition, bacteria in the colon ferment the sugar to produce flatulence and cramping.

Millions of people in the United States have lost the ability to digest lactose, a condition called **lactose intolerance**. Lactose intolerance may be a temporary condition during cancer treatment. If you cannot eat lactose-containing foods, follow the diet in Chapter 25 or supplement the lactase in powder or pill form.

Polysaccharides

Chains of many simple sugars are called **polysaccharides** (*poly* = many). The polysaccharides found in food are starch, dextrin, cellulose, and glycogen.

Half of the carbohydrates we eat are in the form of **starches**. Cooking food softens the cells that contain starch, bursting them and making the starch available to the digestive enzymes of the gastrointestinal tract. Each type of plant produces its own unique type of starch. Each differs by the number of glucose molecules and the arrangement of molecules. Starches can be straight chains of glucose rings or various arrangements of branched chains. They are a time-release form of energy because the glucose made from them enters the bloodstream slowly.

When starches are partially broken down, they form **dextrins**. This can be accomplished by using dry heat (bread in a toaster) or by the action of the digestive enzymes. Dextrins are sweeter than starches and more soluble. Zwieback is a dry, hard bread made from dextrinized starch that is easily digested and is fed to infants. Corn syrup is the partially broken down protein from cornstarch.

Whereas plants store carbohydrate in the form of starch, animals store carbohydrate in a large branched molecule called **glycogen**. It is the most available form of glucose. About three-quarters of a pound of glycogen is stored in the liver and muscles—enough to keep the body fueled for half a day. (However, muscle meat contains very little glycogen when eaten because the glycogen is turned into lactic acid when the animal is slaughtered.) If more carbohydrate is eaten than is needed for immediate use, the remainder is stored as glycogen. When the glycogen capacity of the liver is filled, the rest of the carbohydrate is converted to fat and stored in adipose tissues.

Cellulose is the most abundant organic (carbon-containing) substance on Earth. It forms the structural framework of almost all plants, giving them shape. The glucose units that compose cellulose have a type of bond that resists breakdown by human enzymes. This means that the cellulose from fruits, vegetables, legumes, and grains enters the colon without being digested. Cellulose is the component of fiber that absorbs and holds water, increasing the bulk and softness of the feces.

Fiber

We're told these days that we need **fiber** (roughage or bulk) for a well-functioning digestive tract and to lower risk factors for cancer, heart disease, hypertension, and diabetes. However, no one definition for fiber is totally accepted, nor is it well known how fiber prevents these diseases. A good definition of fiber is a group of carbohydrates or substances made from carbohydrates that show three properties: (1) they resist digestion by human enzymes; (2) they are able to reach the colon in much the same form in which they were eaten; and (3) they have some effect on gastrointestinal function.

Fiber is composed of cellulose, hemicellulose, pectin, algeal substances, gums, and mucilages. **Crude fiber** is a scientific measurement of the cellulose and lignin in a food that is treated with acid and alkali. Estimates of crude fiber are often found in food tables. **Dietary fiber** includes two to five times more substances than crude fiber. It includes cellulose, lignin, hemicelluloses, gums, pectin, and other fibers.

Fiber can be divided into two main subclasses. These are commonly called soluble and insoluble.

Soluble Fiber

As its name suggests, **soluble fiber** is able to dissolve in the watery contents of the digestive tract, where it is thickened into a gel-like consistency. It is easily fermented by the "friendly" bacteria that grow in the colon and is able to affect the entire body.

Soluble fiber reaches the colon without being digested. There it is fermented by bacteria to produce gases (carbon dioxide, hydrogen, and methane), lactic acid, and short-chain fatty acids, mainly acetate, propionate, and butyrate. These fermentation products then interact with the cells of the digestive tract or are absorbed into the bloodstream. Short-chain fatty acids can travel to the liver, where they reduce cholesterol production and influence the metabolism of glucose and fats.

A diet high in soluble fiber is associated with a lower serum cholesterol, lower insulin levels in the blood, and an increased feeling of fullness. Soluble fiber also slows the rate at which food leaves the stomach. Pectin, gums, mucilages, and algeal substances are examples of soluble fiber.

Insoluble Fiber

The other category of fiber, **insoluble fiber**, is not appetizing to the colonic bacteria and leaves the body in much the same form as it entered. Insoluble fiber has a local effect on the digestive tract, increasing size and weight of the feces through water absorption. This increases the frequency of bowel movements, stimulates peristaltic movement, and reduces the time it takes for food to travel through the digestive system. A diet rich in insoluble fiber is associated with a decreased risk of colon and rectal cancer, decreased constipation, and a reduction in blood pressure.

Insoluble fibers are cellulose, hemicellulose, and lignin. **Cellulose** is a form of plant carbohydrate found in fruit and vegetable pulp, skin, stems, and leaves and the outer covering of nuts, seeds, and grains. **Hemicellulose** is a polysaccharide made from hexoses, pentoses, and acid forms of hexoses and pentoses, as well as glucose units. It is found along with cellulose. **Lignin** is a fiber that is not a carbohydrate, although it is found in the cell walls of plants. Sources include wheat bran and woody portions of fruits and vegetables. Lignin is associated with a lower incidence of breast and ovarian cancers.

Alcohol

When yeast ferments the glucose in sugar, fruits, or cereal grains, **ethanol** (a type of alcohol) is produced. Chemically, ethanol is a small, water-soluble molecule that is very easily absorbed. It is metabolized and detoxified in the liver.

Alcohol is a double-edged sword. In some people it causes addiction, and in others it is health promoting. Alcohol can interact with other drugs and alter their effectiveness, so it is very important to tell your doctor how much alcohol you consume each day. Alcohol also puts additional stress on the liver at a time when this important organ needs support. We recommend that you avoid all alcohol during your cancer treatment. If you would like to continue receiving the health benefits of wine, substitute purple grape juice.

Function of Carbohydrates

The body needs a constant supply of carbohydrates in the form of glucose for all metabolic reactions. The energy needs of the body take precedence over all other needs.

The main function of carbohydrate is to provide a source of energy. Each gram of carbohydrate provides approximately four kilocalories (usually used in shortened form, *calorie*) of energy. This is true of both sugars and starches.

Carbohydrates have a protein-sparing effect. This means that if not enough carbohydrates are consumed, the body will then turn to protein as an energy source. For amino acids to be properly absorbed and used, they must be consumed with carbohydrate. Therefore, one way to increase the amount of protein available for new-tissue synthesis is to consume a diet high in carbohydrates.

Carbohydrates are also necessary for normal fat metabolism. If not enough carbohydrates are consumed, the body can also turn to fat for energy. This is the theory behind dieting for weight loss. But the conversion of fat to glucose can go only so fast, and soon the process is starting faster than it can finish. Intermediate products called **ketones** build up and can cause **acidosis** (too much acid in the blood). Sodium combines with these acids, and they are excreted as sodium salts in the urine. This high concentration of sodium in the urine then pulls water into the urine, leading to dehydration and a loss of sodium. The initial weight loss on a very low calorie diet is due to water loss, and the bad breath is due to the excretion of ketones by the lungs.

Glucose is the sole energy source for the brain. Any lack of glucose, or of oxygen to burn the glucose, results in permanent brain damage.

Carbohydrates and their products are precursors of nucleic acids, connective tissue matrix, and galactosides of nerve tissue.

Sugar Red Flags

Sugars often appear on food labels and ingredient lists under different names. Be aware when you see these terms:

Fructose	Maltose
Glucose	Barley malt
High-fructose corn syrup	Brown rice syrup
Sucrose	Honey
Corn syrup	Molasses
Lactose	Fruit juice
Milk sugar	Naturally sweetened
Dextrose	Fruit juice concentrate

In addition, whole foods that are good sources of carbohydrates are also good sources of protein, minerals, and the B vitamins necessary for carbohydrate metabolism.

Metabolism of Carbohydrates

Carbohydrates must be broken down into their component monosaccharides before they can be absorbed. The glucose absorbed through the intestine immediately goes into the portal vein, which transports it to the liver and eventually the bloodstream. As a meal is digested, the amount of blood glucose rises. In response to the glucose in the blood, the pancreas secretes a hormone called **insulin** into the blood. This results in glucose and insulin reaching the hungry cell at the same time.

Glucose cannot enter a cell without insulin. Insulin is like a key that opens the cell door or receptor site. When not enough insulin is secreted, the cells can be surrounded by glucose but unable to use it, since all its doors are locked. This is the dilemma in diabetes, where some of the excess sugar is excreted in the urine, where it can be detected by a urine test.

When the glucose enters a cell, it has several options. If the cell is hungry, the glucose is used immediately to make energy. If the cell is not hungry, the glucose is changed by muscle and liver cells into glycogen for temporary storage. If the storage room for glycogen is filled up, the remaining glucose is changed into fat and stored in regular cells or in the adipose (fat storage) cells.

The next time cells get hungry and no glucose is available from a meal, the glycogen stored in the muscles and liver is changed back into glucose and fed to the cells. When the glycogen is used up, then fat is used to make glucose. This stimulates the appetite, causing you to eat more and make more glucose available. The process of making new glucose is called **gluconeogenesis** (*gluco* = sugar, *neo* = new, *genesis* = to make).

Sometimes when insulin and glucose meet before a hungry cell, they find that there are few doors or receptor sites for the glucose to enter through. This results in **insulin resis-**

tance, also referred to as a decrease in **insulin tolerance**.

Fructose also is absorbed into the portal system. In the liver its atoms are rearranged to form glucose. The liver then releases the glucose when it deems fit.

Carbohydrates and Cancer

Cancer cells in a tumor like to eat glucose and will alter the metabolism of the body to get more. They do this by increasing liver gluconeogenesis from amino acids, which leads to a loss of muscle tissue from the skeleton and internal organs. Insulin resistance is increased so that glucose will not be as able to enter healthy cells. All of this results in **hyperglycemia**, or high blood sugar levels.

One of the purposes of nutrition therapy for cancer is to deny the growing tumor glucose while providing enough for the central nervous system and red blood cell formation. This can be done in a crude way by keeping the blood sugar levels even. You can do this by following these guidelines:

- Avoiding eating or drinking *anything* that tastes sweet on an empty stomach. This includes sweet-tasting fruit and vegetable juices, fruit, soda pop, sweetened refined cereals, honey, or any liquid sweetened with any form of sugar.
- Always eat a balanced meal with mixed foods. A meal rich in complex carbohydrates and fiber will slow the release of food from the stomach, thereby slowing the release of glucose from the meal.
- Eat sweet whole foods such as fruit only with meals. Drink diluted low-sugar fruit and vegetable juices only with fat-containing meals.

A diet in which most of the calories came from unrefined carbohydrates is also rich in many other nutrients that can inhibit the growth of cancer cells.

Summary

Carbohydrates are sugar chains of varying lengths. The body uses them to supply energy for heat and mechanical work, spare protein and fats, feed the healthy colonic bacteria, and provide indigestible fiber for colon health. Whole food rich in complex carbohydrates prevents quick rises in blood glucose that may feed cancerous cells. They are also sources of other cancer-fighting vitamins, minerals, and phytochemicals.

7

···

Lipids, Fats, and Oils

*F*ats are made by animals as a way of storing energy obtained from plants. This energy can be in the guise of preformed fat, carbohydrate, or protein. All fats contain the same number of calories, but not all fats are created equal. This chapter will help you distinguish between healthy fats and those that may promote cancer growth and development.

The word fat gets a lot of bad press. Fat is not a single homogeneous group. Some fats are good, and some are bad. Sometimes it is not the type of fats eaten that causes a problem, but the amount eaten.

The words *fats*, *oils*, and *lipids* are used interchangeably for the same nutrient. Technically fats and oils (which are liquid fats) are part of a group of substances called lipids. In a general sense, **lipids** are organic (carbon-containing) substances that will not dissolve in water.

Other terms that add to the confusion are saturated fats, polyunsaturated fats, omega-3 fats, canola oil, borage oil, monounsaturates, essential fatty acids, nonessential fatty acids, fish oil, olive oil, cholesterol, EPO, EPA, DHA, GLA, and lecithin. These substances, we are told, affect your LDL, HDL, and VLDL. All of these "fat" terms are freely used in conversation today, but few people really understand what they are or what they do. To appreciate the important role lipids play in cancer therapy, a little bit of biochemistry is in order.

Fatty Acids

The basic building block of lipids is the **fatty acid**. Fatty acids are composed of carbon atoms arranged in a chain. At one end of the chain is a methyl group (CH_3), and at the other end is the carboxyl group (COOH). Two smaller fatty acids can be joined together to produce a longer fatty acid by connecting the methyl end of one with the carboxyl group of the other.

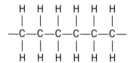

Composition of a fatty acid

The fatty acids that are the building blocks of lipids can be classified according to the degree of saturation, location of the first double bond, and length of the carbon chain.

Saturated and Unsaturated Fatty Acids

Each carbon atom in the carbon chain of a fatty acid has sites for two hydrogen atoms. When the carbon chain of a fatty acid has all the hydrogen atoms it can hold, it is said to be **saturated**. As you can see, the chain of a saturated fatty acid is straight, making it easy for saturated fat molecules to be packed tightly together. This results in a solid fat at room temperature. Saturated fatty acids are very stable and do not go rancid easily. However, many saturated fats increase cholesterol production and blood cholesterol levels. Butter is a natural fat that is high in saturated fatty acids.

Saturated fatty acid chain

When two hydrogen atoms are removed from two adjacent carbon atoms, the carbon atoms use the available sites to add another bond between them, making it a **double**

bond. A fatty acid with one double bond is said to be a **monounsaturated fatty acid** (*mono* = one).

The double bond also causes a kink in the chain. This makes it difficult to stack the chains, just as it is difficult to stack folded chairs on top of one that is partially open. The chains, like the folded chairs, fall around each other; as a result, the fat is a liquid. The greater the percentage of monounsaturated fatty acids in a fat, the more fluid it becomes.

In longer carbon chains, more than one double bond may

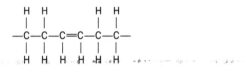

Monounsaturated fatty acid

be formed. These fatty acids are called polyunsaturated fatty acids (*poly* = many). Because polyunsaturated fatty acids have two or more double-bond "kinks," fats that contain a high percentage of polyunsaturates are liquid at room temperature. Polyunsaturates keep the membranes of cells fluid and pliable.

The double bonds in polyunsaturated fatty acids are vul-

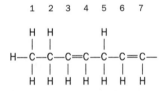

Polyunsaturated fatty acid

nerable to attack from oxygen in the air. The addition of oxygen (oxidation) causes changes in flavor and odor which are commonly called rancidity. Rancid oils can be toxic in large doses. To prevent oxidation in some polyunsaturated fatty acids, hydrogen is added to the double-bonded carbons, breaking the additional bond and making the fatty acid more stable. This is called **hydrogenation**.

Hydrogenated oils are solid at room temperature. The

greater the degree of saturation, the more solid a fat becomes. The lower the saturation, the more liquid it becomes. Tub margarines have a lower degree of saturation than those that come in cubes.

When fatty acids are hydrogenated, they increase the saturation of fats. A high intake of saturated fats is a risk factor for many diseases.

$$-\text{C}=\text{C}- \quad + \quad \text{H}_2 \quad = \quad -\text{C}-\text{C}-$$

unsaturated + hydrogen = hydrogenated fatty acid

Hydrogenation

Omega Number and Length

Another way of classifying fatty acids is by the location of the *first* double bond. This location is found by counting from the methyl end of the molecule. For example, in the preceding figure of a polyunsaturated fatty acid, the first double bond is found on the third carbon. Therefore, its **omega number** is 3. Oils rich in omega-3 fatty acids (in particular, fish oil) are often in the news these days.

Three important omega-3 fatty acids are eicosapentaenoic acid (EPA), docosahexaenoic acid (DHA), and linolenic acid. These fatty acids lower blood triglyceride levels, decrease platelet stickiness, and keep the arteries clean from fatty deposits. How this is done is not well understood. However, to get the most of these fats, eat fish with the skin on (unlike chicken, which should be eaten with the skin removed). The body can manufacture EPA and DHA from linolenic acid, but it does not always manufacture enough. By adding supplemental EPA and DHA through fish oil, you can enjoy the benefits of these fatty acids.

The omega-6 fatty acids also have unique properties. They include linoleic acid, which the body cannot manufacture but must obtain from the diet; arachidonic acid, which is manufactured from linoleic acid; and gamma linolenic acid (GLA). GLA is manufactured as a result of the first step toward the production of hormone-like substances called prostaglandins. Not everyone manufactures enough GLA; those who do not can benefit from supplements. Good sources of GLA are evening primrose oil and borage tree oil.

Chain Length
Fatty acids are also described by the length of their carbon chain. Formic acid (released in bee stings and ant bites) has only one carbon atom. Acetic acid (vinegar) has two carbon atoms. Since these fatty acids are so short, they are soluble in water, making them act more like water-soluble acids. The fatty acids found in food range from four carbons (butyric acid) to twenty-four (found in fish oils).

Within this range, fatty acids are described as having short, medium, or long chains:
- Short-chain fatty acids contain two to six carbon atoms. They are found in butter and milk.
- Medium-chain fatty acids contain eight to twelve carbon atoms. These are very easy to absorb and are available at pharmacies as medium-chain triglycerides (MCTs). Coconut is very rich in MCTs.
- Long-chain fatty acids contain 16 or more carbon atoms.

Applying the Classifications: An Example
Let's see how we would classify the molecule pictured. We know it is a fatty acid because it follows the formula of a methyl group at one end, a carboxyl group at the other, and two to twenty carbons in between. It has three double bonds, so it is a polyunsaturated fatty acid. With eighteen carbon atoms, it is a long chain fatty acid. Double bonds are at carbon numbers 3, 6, and 9, so its omega number is 3.

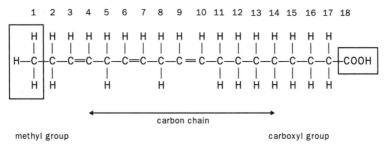

Linolenic acid

This fatty acid has a *cis-* configuration; both the hydrogens on the double-bonded carbons are on the same side of the molecule. *Cis-* and *trans-* are descriptions of the arrangement of hydrogen atoms around the double bonds. The *cis-*configuration is the one that occurs in nature.

This may seem a trivial point, but the shape of a molecule determines its function. Alter the shape, alter the function. Molecules that are *trans-* versions do not have the same effect in the body as the natural *cis-* version. This has been demonstrated with *trans-* fatty acids found in margarines and spreads. They may elevate cholesterol just as much as, if not more than, saturated fats.

Essential Fatty Acids

The body can manufacture all of the fatty acids it needs except for the **essential fatty acids (EFAS)**. There are two EFAS: linoleic acid and linolenic acid. (The preceding example was a representation of linolenic acid.) Since the body cannot manufacture EFAS, they must be obtained from the diet.

Both EFAS are precursors to prostaglandins. By varying the ratio of EFAS, it is possible to manipulate prostaglandin synthesis.

Young children need more EFAS than adults, and males need more than females. Children under two years that are fed low-fat cows' milk can develop an EFA deficiency.

Types of Lipids

How are fatty acids related to the everyday fats and oils we
are familiar with? In general, they combine to form lipids
(fats) in food.

Triglycerides

Most of the lipids in foods are **triglycerides**, combinations
of four molecules: the glycerol molecule, which acts as a
three- "rod" hanger, and the three fatty acids that hang from
each "rod." The properties and abilities of each triglyceride
depend upon the characteristics of its component fatty acids.

For example, the properties of an oil are related to the
types of triglycerides found in that oil. In turn, the proper-

```
        H                                H
        |                                |
     H—C—OH                       H—C—OOC—R1
        |                                |
   OH—C—H   + 3(R—COOH)  =  R2—COO—C—C
        |                                |
     H—C—OH                       H—C—OOC—R3
        |                                |
        H                                H

   Glycerol  + 3 fatty acids  =        triglyceride
```

Formation of a triglyceride

ties of triglycerides are determined by the fatty acids that
form it, and the properties of the fatty acids are determined
by their structure. The longer and more unsaturated the fatty
acids, the more liquid or soft the fat is at room temperature.
The order of the fatty acids on the glycerol molecule also
affect the digestibility and absorbability of the triglyceride.
Because so many different fatty acids are present in natural
foods, many types of triglycerides are found in a fat or oil.

Besides triglycerides, foods also contain **monoglycerides**
(with one fatty acid hanging on the glycerol) and **diglycerides** (with two fatty acid molecules). These molecules are
also produced during the digestion of triglycerides.

Sterols

Another familiar group of lipids is the sterols, with the most infamous sterol being **cholesterol**. Cholesterol is found only in animal foods and is manufactured in the liver. Not all bad, it is the precursor for steroids, including bile acids and the sex hormones. In the liver it can be converted to the precursor of vitamin D, it waterproofs the skin, and it is necessary for proper brain development in infants. **Beta sitosterol**, found in rice bran, competes with cholesterol for absorption, so it reduces blood cholesterol levels.

Compound Lipids

The final group of lipids consists of the following members:

- **Phospholipids** are compounds of fatty acids, phosphoric acid, and a nitrogen-containing base. One of the most common phospholipids is lecithin.
- **Glycolipids** are compounds of fatty acids, carbohydrate, and a nitrogen-containing base. Glycolipids are part of nerve tissue and certain cell membranes.
- **Sulpholipids** are lipids that contain sulfur.
- **Lipoproteins** are lipids combined with protein. Well-known lipoproteins include **chylomicrons,** the form in which lipids are packaged to travel in the lymph system to the bloodstream; **very low density lipoproteins (VLDLS)**, the transport packages for triglycerides in the blood; **low-density lipoproteins (LDLS)**, the package that carries cholesterol to the tissues and is commonly referred to as "bad" cholesterol; and **high-density lipoproteins (HDLS)**,the "good" cholesterol that removes cholesterol from the tissues and brings it back to the liver.
- **Lipopolysaccharides** are lipids that contain polysaccharides.

Storage of Lipids

Humans have two types of body fat: brown fat and white fat. Most fat is white. It is made of adipose cells that accumulate beneath the skin, around internal organs, and inside muscle tissue. These fat cells store fat as liquid triglycerides.

Brown adipose tissue occurs in much smaller amounts. It decreases with age and is involved in thermogenesis, the response to cold. Brown fat produces energy in the form of heat, warming the body.

Function of Lipids

Although we have a tendency to consider lipids bad, they are necessary for human life. Their functions include the following:

- Fats are the most concentrated form of energy. They provide nine calories for every gram burned, which is more than twice the amount of energy per gram of carbohydrate.
- Adipose (fat) tissue holds organs in place, and the subcutaneous (below the skin) layer of fat provides insulation from the cold and maintains body temperature.
- Fat spares the B vitamin thiamine. Thiamine is required when using carbohydrate for energy.
- Fat spares protein. When fat is present, the body does not have to burn protein for fuel.
- Fat helps in the absorption and transport of the fat-soluble vitamins A, D, E, and K.
- Lipids slow the rate at which foods leave the stomach. This means that the carbohydrate also present is not released all at once, keeping insulin and blood sugar levels even. Fat decreases the appetite, giving the feeling of satiety.
- Fat makes foods more palatable.
- Lipids provide the building blocks from which sterols,

prostaglandins, thromboxanes, prostacyclins, and cell membranes are made.

Metabolism of Lipids

Fat molecules are too large to be absorbed directly and must be broken down into smaller units. The enzymes responsible for lipid digestion are called **lipases** (*lipo* = fat, *-ase* = enzyme). Gastric lipase (*gastric* = stomach) partially emulsifies and digests the short- and medium-chain fatty acids, and many are absorbed before they have a chance to reach the small intestine.

When fats are detected in the duodenum, bile made in the liver is secreted into the small intestine. Bile is an emulsifying agent. It breaks down fat into small lipid droplets in the same way shampoo emulsifies the oils in your hair. In this way lipids, mainly long-chain fatty acids, are more accessible to the lipases secreted by the pancreas. They are digested to produce monoglycerides, diglycerides, and free fatty acids, which are absorbed into the intestinal wall and then reassembled on the other side into triglycerides.

These triglycerides are packaged into lipoprotein droplets called **chylomicrons** for transport by the lymphatic system, bypassing the portal vein that takes the water-soluble compounds to the liver. Lymph vessels bring them to the left shoulder, where they are discharged into the bloodstream. Chylomicrons are large enough to make plasma look "milky" after a fat-rich meal.

Medium-chain triglycerides (MCTs)—those with a chain of eight to ten carbons—need very little lipase and no bile to be digested. Unlike the long chains, they do not need to be reassembled into triglycerides after absorption. They easily dissolve into the blood and are carried via the portal vein to the liver. Because they bypass the slow-moving lymph system, MCTs are absorbed as fast as glucose. They are an excellent source of energy for cancer patients who have damage to their intestinal villi due to malnutrition, radiation, or chemotherapy or those who lack sufficient pancreatic enzymes or bile acids.

Pure MCT in oil form can be purchased in pharmacies without a prescription. It is not very palatable and must be mixed with other foods. Coconut milk is a good source of palatable MCTS.

Cancer and Lipids

Too much fat in the diet is linked with increased tumor growth. This may be the result of fats stimulating the multiplication and spread of cancer cells, fats inhibiting the immune system, or both.

Linoleic and linolenic acid, the essential fatty acids, differ in their ability to promote cancer. Linoleic acid is a precursor of arachidonic acid, an omega-6 fatty acid, which is a precursor for the prostaglandin E2 series (PGE2). PGE2 reduces the ability of macrophages and natural killer (NK) cells to kill cancer cells and tumors. Linolenic acid inhibits the omega-6 fatty acids by competing for the same enzymes. This means that there is less PGE2 and more prostaglandin E1. When EPA in the form of fish oil is added to the diet, it can also increase PGE1.

The total amount of fat in the diet is important. NK cell activity is increased when fat intake is decreased to 25 percent calories from fat. For those with hormone-dependent cancers such as breast cancer, a very low fat diet (less than 20 percent calories from fat) may slow the spread of cancer cells.

The type of fat in the diet is also important. Most of it should come from oils rich in monounsaturated fatty acids, such as olive and canola oil. This should be accompanied by a low intake of linoleic acid. People with hormone related cancers probably should not supplement omega-6 fatty acids (including evening primrose oil).

Summary

Lipids include dietary fats and oils. The health properties of an oil are determined by the number of double bonds, the location of the first double bond, and the chain length. Fatty acids with only one double bond are health promoting, while fatty acids without double bonds are not. The two essential fatty acids, linolenic and linoleic acid, can be manipulated to increase or decrease prostaglandin synthesis. Diets that contain more linolenic acid than linoleic acid help the immune system in its fight against cancer.

8

....

Protein and Cancer

*P*roteins provide the amino acid building blocks your body needs to build new tissue and repair damaged tissue. In order to quickly repair damage done by cancer treatment, good sources of protein must be eaten each day. The concept of what a good protein is has changed in the last ten years. This chapter will help to update your knowledge as to which sources of protein should be eaten and which should be avoided.

While fats and carbohydrates often suffer from bad press, protein has no such problem. In the public mind, protein is still the most important macronutrient. It is synonymous with strength, victory, and very large muscles. Its name reflects this privileged status. The word *protein* comes from the Greek word meaning "of first importance." In reality, protein must share the spotlight with fats and carbohydrates. No one macronutrient is more important than any other.

Like carbohydrates and lipids, protein is made up of carbon, oxygen, and hydrogen atoms. Protein differs from them in that it also contains a nitrogen atom. Protein is the major structural molecule of the body. Twenty to thirty pounds of an adult's total weight is protein, with half of that being found in the muscles.

All enzymes are proteins. Many hormones are proteins. The only constituents of the body that do not contain protein are urine and bile. Proteins are made up of chains of **amino acids** (*amine* = nitrogen-containing).

Protein Molecule Shape

Twenty-two different amino acids are present in the human body. Each amino acid is joined to the other by means of a **peptide bond** forming **peptide** or **polypeptide chains**. Chemically each amino acid is composed of an amino group, a carboxyl group (*oxyl* = contains oxygen), a hydrogen atom, and the remainder of the molecule, R, which differentiates it from other types. The R group can range in size from twenty-three amino groups to several hundred thousand amino groups.

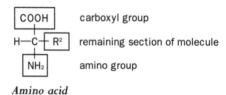

Amino acid

The twenty-two amino acids identified in the body form a sort of alphabet. Each amino acid "letter" can be used to make up an unlimited number of protein words.

What your body does with the protein is determined by the shape of the protein. Chains of polypeptides are twisted together to form a coil that resembles a Slinky toy. The hydrogen atoms in the Slinky form an effective but weak bond between turns of the coil. As long as the hydrogen bonds are intact, the protein holds its coil shape. These coils are then arranged into a specific shape that determines what the body uses it for.

Simple but long arrangements are called **fibrous proteins**. Fibrous proteins are used to make structural parts of tissue, including the collagen in connective tissue, the keratin in hair and nails, and the myosin in muscles. Fibrous proteins do not dissolve in water and are very strong structurally.

If the chain is twisted after it forms a Slinky, it folds into itself, forming a kind of knot. In a peptide coil this knot is held in place by the sulfur-to-sulfur bonds found in some of the amino acids. Slinky knots are called **globular proteins**. Globular proteins form enzymes and are present in the extracellular fluid of plants and animals. They dissolve easily in water. This is the kind of protein found in egg whites, the casein of milk, the hemoglobin of red blood cells, and the albumins and globulins of blood plasma.

When a protein enters the digestive tract, it cannot be absorbed until it has been broken down into its amino acid components. This is done by **hydrolysis**, or the breakage of peptide bonds by the addition of a molecule of water. This produces smaller proteins: individual amino acids, dipeptides

$$H-N-C-C \cdots \cdots \cdots N-C-C-OH$$

$$H_2O$$

Formation of a peptide bond

$$H-N-C-C+OH \quad H+N-C-C-OH$$

$$H_2O$$

Hydrolysis (breakage of a peptide bond)

(two amino acid proteins), and tripeptides (three amino acid proteins), which are easily absorbed by the digestive tract. (Conversely, a peptide bond is formed by removing a molecule of water from two adjacent amino acids.)

The peptide bond can be easily attacked by the digestive enzymes of bacteria. The bacterial growth and formation of potentially toxic proteins as a by-product are the cause of food spoilage. This is why protein foods such as milk, eggs, meat, poultry, and fish must be refrigerated.

Types of Amino Acids

The Nonessential Amino Acids

alanine	hydroxyglutamic acid
arginine	hydroxyproline
aspartic acid	norleucine
citrulline	proline
cystine	serine
glutamic acid	tyrosine
glycine	

Essential Amino Acids

histidine	phenylalanine
isoleucine	threonine
leucine	tryptophan
lysine	valine
methionine	

Essential and Nonessential Amino Acids

The body can manufacture most of the amino acids it needs from carbohydrate, fat, and other amino acids. These are called **nonessential amino acids**. This is a somewhat inaccurate term, since the nonessential amino acids are essential for life. They are nonessential only in the sense they do not have to be obtained from the diet.

Eleven other amino acids cannot be manufactured in amounts needed to support growth and maintenance. These are the **essential amino acids**, and they must be obtained from the diet. Without them, protein cannot be made and body tissues cannot be maintained.

Functions of Amino Acids

Besides forming the building blocks of protein, each amino acid has other specific functions in the body. **Tryptophan** is a precursor of (used to make) niacin, a B vitamin, and serotonin, a neurotransmitter in the brain. **Methionine** provides sulfur groups for protein manufacture and detoxification of toxins by the liver. **Phenylalanine** is a precursor of the amino acid **tyrosine**, used to make hair and skin pigment. **Histidine** is used to make **histamine**, a chemical that dilates blood vessels, and **glycine**, which combines with toxic chemicals and makes them harmless. **Glutamic acid** is a precursor of **gamma-aminobutyric acid (GABA)**, a neurotransmitter.

Complete and Incomplete Proteins

The concept of "complete" and "incomplete" protein is one of the most confusing notions in nutrition. It was developed in an age when animal protein was considered the gold standard of protein quality. Today the ideas of complete and incomplete protein have taken on an entirely new meaning.

The so-called complete proteins contain all nine of the essential amino acids in sufficient quantities to allow growth in a young animal. Not surprisingly, ovalbumin, the main protein in egg, and casein, the main protein in milk, are complete proteins. The protein found in animal flesh is also complete. In the unlikely event that you are dependent on only a single food for survival, it would have to be a complete protein source. This condition, however, rarely occurs except in infancy.

The amino acids obtained from the diet are combined in the body with amino acids recycled from internal tissue breakdown. It is from this amino acid pool that the tissues draw their protein for new cells. The notion of protein combining—the belief that complementary proteins must be eaten at the same meal or a protein deficiency will ensue—has been thoroughly disproven.

Complete proteins also come packaged with "complete fats." Since saturated fat is an absolute necessity for infant brain development and growth, complete-protein foods are likely to be excellent sources of unneeded artery-clogging saturated fats.

Incomplete proteins, on the other hand, lack these saturated fats. Like the complete proteins they contain all nine of the essential amino acids. The only difference is that the amounts of these amino acids differ from food to food, much in the same way vitamin and mineral levels vary.

Incomplete protein sources are superior to complete protein sources. Plant proteins are usually low in total fat and saturated fat; they are free of cholesterol. The high-fat sources of incomplete protein, such as nuts and seeds, contain heart-healthy fats that combat tumor spread. They are also excellent sources of cancer-fighting fiber, minerals, vitamins, and phytochemicals.

Nitrogen Balance

True protein deficiencies are very rare and do not occur in the healthy, well-nourished individual. Protein-calorie malnutrition is a condition due to lack of enough food to maintain health. This can result from much higher than normal protein needs or because of an inability to absorb the protein that is eaten.

Nitrogen balance is a term you are likely to hear used by your physician or nutritionist. Since protein is the only nitrogen-containing macronutrient, the amount of nitrogen in the body is an accurate method of determining protein content of the body. When the amount of protein present in the diet is known and the amount of protein being excreted is known, then the amount of protein left in the body can be measured.

When nitrogen intake and nitrogen output are equal, that individual is said to be in nitrogen balance or equilibrium. This is the usual state for healthy adults.

If an individual has more nitrogen coming in than going out, that person is said to be in positive nitrogen balance. This means the buildup of tissue is greater than the breakdown of tissue. This occurs in pregnant and lactating women; growing infants, children, and adolescents; and adults who are recovering from an illness that resulted in a protein loss.

A negative nitrogen balance indicates the opposite is happening; more nitrogen is leaving than is coming in. The rate of tissue breakdown is greater than the rate of tissue synthesis. This occurs when the body is not taking in enough protein, protein is being burned for energy because not enough fat and carbohydrates are present for fuel, and the protein needs of the body are greatly increased, as in cancer.

Cancer and Protein

The cancer cells change the metabolism of protein so that more amino acids are available for tumor growth. This can translate into a loss of muscle tissue and predisposes cancer patients to a state of negative nitrogen balance.

Most of the protein in your diet should come from plant sources. Plant proteins come complete with numerous cancer-fighting nutrients and phytochemicals. The proteins from fatty fish come packaged with the omega-3 fatty acids necessary for the body's defense system. They should provide the second highest amount of protein in your diet. Skinless poultry should make the smallest contribution to your amino acid pool. Poultry is a good source of minerals but often tastes "wrong" from the effects of chemotherapy and radiation.

Summary

Proteins are composed of amino acids and are the body's only source of nitrogen. They contribute to the formation of body tissues, enzymes, antibodies, hemoglobin, and hormones. Cancer interferes with protein metabolism by burning some of the body's proteins for fuel even when enough carbohydrates and fat are present. A lack of protein has a devastating effect on the immune system.

9

....

Water-Soluble
Vitamins and Cancer

*W*hen nutrition was a young science, researchers found that a synthetic diet of carbohydrate, lipids, proteins, water, and minerals was not enough to allow animals to grow and thrive. This led to the discovery of a group of unrelated carbon-containing compounds called vitamins. Human growth and development requires thirteen vitamins. For classification purposes, they are divided into two groups: those that dissolve in water and those that dissolve in fat. This chapter explores the water-soluble vitamins, their relationship to cancer growth, and ways they can aid in cancer treatment.

The word *vitamin* was coined in 1912 by Casimir Funk. Originally vitamins were recognized only for their ability to prevent deficiency diseases. For example, vitamin C was discovered because of its ability to cure scurvy. With time this definition has proved too narrow. Vitamins are now known to serve many functions in the body besides preventing specific deficiency diseases. For example, many vitamins are also potent antioxidants, and some vitamins enhance absorption of other vitamins or minerals. At the same time, knowledge about vitamin deficiency has broadened to include the following associations with cancer:

- Deficiency of choline or B vitamins leads to increased risk of liver cancer.
- Vitamin E deficiency leads to an overall increased risk of cancer and leukemia.
- Vitamin A deficiency is an overall cancer risk.

- Deficiency of pyridoxine (vitamin B_6) is associated with cervical cancer.

In the United States, the National Research Council establishes dietary standards in terms of **Recommended Dietary Allowances (RDAS)**. When looking at an RDA, keep in mind that the levels are set only to prevent deficiency diseases. For example, the recommendation for vitamin C is set at a level that prevents scurvy. It does not take into account the use of vitamin C as an antioxidant.

Your cell citizens obtain vitamins in three ways:

1. They can absorb vitamins from foods in the digestive tract.
2. Some bacterias in the colon produce vitamins (such as vitamin K), and these can also be absorbed.
3. The body is able to manufacture some vitamins, such as vitamin D.

Vitamins do not provide energy or contribute to cell mass. They prefer to be "the molecules behind the nutrients," so to speak—helper elements that enable other nutrients from the sidelines.

Each individual vitamin is actually a family of related compounds, including precursors and bound forms. Some substances, such as choline, carnitine, inositol, taurine, and pyrroloquinoline quinone, have vitamin-like properties and may be required at particular stages of growth.

Vitamins that can dissolve in water are called water soluble. They includes the B complex vitamins and vitamin C. Water-soluble vitamins are absorbed into the bloodstream via the portal system and brought immediately to the liver before distribution to the body. The body does not store water-soluble vitamins. To keep optimal levels of these nutrients in blood circulation, you need to eat their food sources frequently. Most of the B vitamins function as parts of enzymes. All can be excreted in the urine.

> ## How to Supplement the B Vitamins
>
> If a supplement is necessary, take a balanced B complex. If you are allergic or sensitive to yeast, look for a yeast-free supplement.
>
> Always take a B complex supplement on a full stomach. Otherwise stomach irritation can occur. You will know if the supplement is being absorbed if your urine takes on a bright yellow color.
>
> Do not buy a time-release B complex supplement. Each B vitamin is absorbed in a different area of the gastrointestinal tract. The vitamins released past their absorption point will be lost in the feces.
>
> If you need to supplement only one particular B vitamin, also take a B complex supplement as a base.
>
> Very large doses of some B vitamins can cause liver damage. Have your health care provider perform regular liver function tests.

The B Complex Vitamins

The B complex vitamins are known for two major functions: First, they are an absolute necessity for the conversion of carbohydrate into glucose, the body's main energy source. Second, they are essential for the proper functioning of the nervous system. In addition, the B vitamins help to strengthen cellular membranes, fortifying them against stress.

The B complex vitamins share a close relationship. A deficiency in one may impair the use of the others, and supplementation of one may cause a deficiency in the others. That is why the B complex should be considered one vitamin rather than a group of single nutrients. Never take megadoses of one particular B vitamin without medical supervision.

Like the other water-soluble vitamins, the B vitamins are not stored in large amounts. This has been misinterpreted to mean that excess will "wash away" in the urine. Like all substances, the B vitamins must be detoxified before the kidney can excrete them.

Sources of B vitamins include brewer's yeast (nutritional yeast), whole grains and cereals, wheat and rice bran and germ, beans, nuts and seeds, milk, eggs, and leafy green vegetables.

Thiamine, or Vitamin B₁

During absorption, thiamine is converted to thiamine pyrophosphate. In this active form, thiamine is involved with energy production and nerve maintenance and conduction. Thiamine is lost when grains are refined. Deficiency can cause a lack of appetite, irritability, fatigue, depression, sleep disorders, and weight loss.

Sources of thiamine include brewer's yeast, almonds, wheat germ, nuts, beans, whole grains, split peas, mung beans, and lentils.

Riboflavin, Riboflavin Phosphate, or Vitamin B₂

Riboflavin is a critical part of flavin mononucleotide and flavin adenine dinucleotide, coenzymes involved in energy production. The production of these enzymes from riboflavin can be affected by hormones and drugs. Thyroid hormones and adrenal steroids enhance their production, and tricyclic antidepressants and phenothiazines inhibit their production.

The need for riboflavin increases with energy intake and growth needs. When B complex is taken as a food supplement, the breakdown products of riboflavin give the urine a bright yellow color and pungent odor.

Sources of riboflavin include brewer's yeast, almonds, wheat germ, wild rice, mushrooms, millet, mackerel, soybeans, eggs, and split peas.

Niacin, Nicotinamide, or Nicotinic Acid

Niacin is an essential component of nicotinamide adenine dinucleotide and nicotinamide adenine dinucleotide phosphate, coenzymes needed for metabolism. It is absorbed from the diet and can also be manufactured by the body from the amino acid tryptophan.

Niacin is available in a time-release form that does not cause the "flushing" effect seen in regular supplements. This time-release form, however, has been linked to liver damage, so it should never be taken in high doses or for prolonged periods.

Sources of niacin include brewer's yeast, wheat bran, peanuts, sunflower and sesame seeds, pine nuts, brown rice, and seed oils.

Pyridoxine, Pyridoxal, Pyridoxamine, or Vitamin B_6

In the tissues, all forms of vitamin B_6 are converted to pyridoxal 5-phosphate, a coenzyme needed for fat and protein metabolism and immune functioning. Pyridoxal 5-phosphate is necessary for the proper metabolism of the amino acid tryptophan. It is a necessary part of over 100 enzyme systems.

Vitamin B_6 is necessary for the immune system, where it is involved in antibody production. A deficiency of pyridoxine reduces the number of disease-fighting lymphocytes and lowers the ability of other immune elements to respond to the chemical messengers sent by the lymphocytes.

Food processing can destroy some of the B_6 present in foods. Pregnancy, lactation, an overactive thyroid, or a high intake of animal protein can cause a need for extra B_6.

Sources of pyridoxine include brewer's yeast, sunflower seeds, wheat germ, tuna, beans, salmon, trout, mackerel, brown rice, bananas, halibut, walnuts, hazelnuts, avocados, egg yolks, and kale.

Folic Acid, Folacin, Folate, Tetrahydrofolic Acid

Folic acid is the commonly used term for pteroyl-polyglutamic acid, the precursor of a large family of folate compounds. It is needed for RNA synthesis. A deficiency of this vitamin causes megoblastic anemia and has been associated with a degeneration of the intestinal lining, which then further reduces nutrient absorption. Folic acid may help block dysplasia, a condition where cells that have begun to divide rapidly may become malignant. Even a mild folic acid deficiency may promote cervical dysplasia.

The body cannot make any folate and therefore must obtain all it needs from the diet. Folates are very sensitive to heat. Boiling, steaming, or frying for five to ten minutes may destroy up to 96 percent of the folate in a food.

Sources of folic acid include brewer's yeast, black-eyed peas, wheat and rice germ and bran, beans, soy foods, lentils, asparagus, leafy green vegetables, green cruciferous vegetables, whole wheat, oatmeal, barley, almonds, walnuts, and split peas.

Vitamin B_{12}, or Cobalamin

In the stomach, cobalamin is released from its dietary sources by peptic digestion. Cells in the stomach lining produce a substance called intrinsic factor (IF), which binds to the vitamin, forming an IF-cobalamin complex. This complex is resistant to digestion and is readily absorbed in the small intestine.

Vitamin B_{12} is involved in protein, fat, and carbohydrate metabolism. Older people do not always produce enough intrinsic factor, making absorption difficult. Microorganisms are the ultimate source of all vitamin B_{12} in the diet. Strict vegans may have to supplement this nutrient.

Sources of vitamin B_{12} include shellfish, fish, egg yolks, skinless poultry, yogurt, and milk.

Biotin

Biotin is essential for many enzyme systems. It is present in most foods and can be made by intestinal bacteria and absorbed from there. It is resistant to heat and related metabolically to B_{12}, folate, and pantothenic acid.

Sources of biotin include mushrooms, egg yolks, bananas, grapefruit, watermelon, and strawberries.

Pantothenic Acid

A part of coenzyme A, pantothenic acid is involved in the release of energy from carbohydrate and in the breakdown and use of fatty acids. It also reduces stress. Milling cereal grains reduces their content of pantothenic acid by 50 percent.

Sources of pantothenic acid include eggs, salmon, whole-grain cereals, legumes, brewer's yeast, cauliflower, broccoli, potatoes, tomatoes, and molasses.

Vitamin C, or Ascorbic Acid

Perhaps the most famous and favorite vitamin is vitamin C. It is the antioxidant responsible for protecting the watery parts of the cell from free radical damage. Vitamin C prevents the oxidation of folate, thereby increasing the amount of folate available to the body. It enhances the absorption of iron and the bioavailablity of stored iron. For example, when a vitamin C source such as orange juice is eaten with a slice of whole wheat bread, the iron in the bread becomes free for absorption. Humans are among the few mammals unable to make their own vitamin C. Most other mammals are able to manufacture their own supplies as needed.

Vitamin C detoxifies histamine, which can suppress the immune system. It helps build dense connective tissue, which may inhibit tumor invasion, and research shows it enhances antibiotic therapy. The emotional and physical stress of having cancer may increase your body's use of vitamin C.

How to Supplement Vitamin C

Ascorbic acid is very easily lost to the urine, so avoid taking the recommended dose all at once. This will cause the blood levels of vitamin C to rise and then plummet. Take vitamin C in smaller doses throughout the day, or buy a time-release capsule or sustained-release tablet.

For best absorption, take vitamin C with food. Consider taking a form of vitamin C that includes the bioflavonoids. These work synergistically with vitamin C.

Sources of vitamin C include sweet peppers, kale, collard and turnip greens, broccoli, strawberries, papaya, citrus fruits, mangoes, cantaloupe, and cabbage.

Summary

Vitamins are organic compounds that serve as helpers to other nutrients in the biochemical processes of digestion, absorption, and metabolism. There are two types: water soluble and fat soluble. The water-soluble vitamins are vitamin C, thiamine, riboflavin, niacin, pyridoxine, folacin, cobalamin, biotin, and pantothenic acid.

These vitamins are particularly vulnerable to light, heat, and air. Therefore, fresh, raw fruits and vegetables have higher concentrations of the water-soluble vitamins than cooked or aged produce.

10

Fat-Soluble
Vitamins and Cancer

*F*at-soluble vitamins are intimately related to lipids. They need fat to be absorbed, and when cancer treatment interferes with fat absorption, a deficiency of these vitamins may occur. This chapter explains how the fat-soluble vitamins protect healthy tissues while enhancing the strength of the immune army.

There are four families of fat-soluble vitamins: vitamin A, vitamin D, vitamin E, and vitamin K. These vitamins need to be dissolved in fat before they can be absorbed in the intestine. Low-fat and low-calorie diets, whether by chance or by purpose, risk not providing enough of these vitamins.

Dietary fats and the fat-soluble vitamins are absorbed into the lymph vessels, bypassing the portal blood system that takes water-soluble nutrients to the liver. After a long climb up to your shoulder, they are dumped into the left subclavian artery.

Vitamins A and D can be toxic in large amounts when taken over a long period. They are stored in fatty tissues and the liver, and they can accumulate over time. Unlike vitamin C and the B complex, the fat-soluble vitamins are very stable. They are better able to stand up to the heat of cooking and processing.

Vitamin A, Retinol, Retinal, Retinoic Acid, Retinyl Esters

The vitamin A or retinoid family contains several forms, natural and synthetic, that have vitamin A activity. In addition, a number of vegetable foods contain compounds that the body can convert into vitamin A, such as the alpha, beta, and gamma carotenes. Absorption of retenol requires bile, pancreatic enzymes, and antioxidants. In the form of retinoic acid, it is absorbed directly. A six-month supply of vitamin A is stored in the liver as retinyl esters.

Vitamin A can be toxic in dosages over 15,000 RE, but much of this toxicity can be prevented by also taking vitamin E. Vitamin E and vitamin A work together.

Vitamin A can promote differentiation in epithelial cells and regression of premalignant lesions. It inhibits the development of cancerous tumors. A lack of vitamin A will decrease antibody formation, while vitamin A supplementation increases cytotoxic action of T cells, NK cells, and macrophages.

Vitamin D, Cholecalciferol (D_3), Ergosterol (D_2), Calcitriol

The vitamin D family has two possible sources: preformed from the diet and synthesized by the skin. Vitamin D is called the sunshine vitamin, because the large amounts of the precursor 7-dehydrocholesterol in the skin, when exposed to the ultraviolet light from the sun, are converted into cholecalciferol (vitamin D_3). It is estimated that up to 80 percent of the body's needs for vitamin D can be obtained this way. How much is produced depends on how much melanin pigment is in the skin (melanin competes with the precursor for the light), how much skin is exposed, and how much sun reaches the skin. This means that dark-skinned people who live in cold climates (reducing skin area open to sun) and any people who live in low-sun areas (Seattle or England, for example) probably cannot rely on manufacturing enough of their own vitamin D. The elderly are also at risk, since they often cannot get out and do not eat fortified foods.

Vitamin D is a hormone that regulates mineral balance. It stimulates intestinal absorption of calcium and phosphorus, works with the parathyroid hormone to mobilize calcium from bone, and stimulates the reabsorption of calcium from the kidneys. It also plays a role in cellular differentiation and development.

Sources of vitamin D include sunshine, fortified cows' milk and soymilk, deep-sea fish and fish oils, and egosterol in plants.

Tips for Using Supplements

When purchasing fat-soluble vitamins and supplements, be sure they are fresh. If the supplements are past pull date or close to the date on the bottles, do not purchase them. Oils must be very fresh to neutralize free radicals. Rancid oils—ones that smell fishy or like Play-Doh—are old, inactive, and can cause more free radicals in the body. Store oils and fat-soluble supplements in the refrigerator, inside airtight containers. Keep them out of direct sunlight as much as possible.

Vitamin E, Tocopherol, Tocotrienol

The vitamin E family is a group of eight closely related fat-soluble compounds made up of four tocopherols (alpha, beta, delta, gamma) and four tocotrienols. Vitamin E is stored in all areas of the body in fatty deposits, the liver, and the muscle. Eating a lot of linoleic acid and polyunsaturated fatty acids decreases the amount of vitamin E absorbed by reducing the micelle formation which is necessary for absorption. Vitamin E is an antioxidant. It works in partnership with vitamin C, protecting the lipids in the cell as vitamin C protects the watery contents. It protects vitamins A, C, and the carotenes from oxidation.

Vitamin E may protect healthy cells from some of the toxicity of radiation therapy and decrease the toxicity of certain chemotherapy drugs. It also appears to stimulate the immune system and protect the lipids in the cell membrane from damage.

Sources of vitamin E include wheat germ oil, germ of cereals, egg yolk, and nuts.

Vitamin K, Phylloquinone (K₁), Menaquinone (K₂), Menadione (Synthetic Form of K₃)

Vitamin K_1 is found in green plants, while vitamin K_2 is produced by bacteria in the colon. In the liver vitamin K acts as a coenzyme in reactions that produce the clotting factors and can interfere with the anticlotting effects of anticoagulants. However at doses lower than one milligram per day, Vitamin K_1 does not pose a threat and may actually enhance the antimetastatic effects of anticoagulants.

Vitamin K may also act as a toxin to cancer cells while not harming normal cells.

Sources of vitamin K include cabbage, broccoli, turnip greens, lettuce, wheat bran, cheese, and egg yolk.

Summary

The four fat-soluble vitamin families, A, D, E, and K, are often depleted in cancer patients. This is usually caused by fat malabsorption. These vitamins are often difficult to obtain in the diet, and a low-dose supplement can be very helpful in rebuilding stores. Vitamin E is a nontoxic antioxidant that protects the other fat-soluble vitamins and oils from oxidation. It can be taken in larger doses and should always accompany any supplemented oils (such as flaxseed or fish oil), and the other fat-soluble vitamins.

11

Minerals and Cancer

$\mathcal{M}$inerals are the elements in simple inorganic form. Mineral elements that the body needs in large amounts are called the macrominerals. Those needed in small amounts are called the trace minerals, and those needed in minute amounts the ultra trace minerals. Over twenty-two minerals are considered to be essential, with more identified as science progresses. This chapter describes the role of minerals in the diet, especially for people with cancer.

Minerals may take the form of ions (atoms that carry an electrical charge) or salts. Metals form positive ions (**cations**), and nonmetals form negative ions (**anions**). Metal cations include sodium, potassium, magnesium, and calcium. Nonmetal anions include chlorine (chloride), sulfur (sulfate), phosphorus (phosphate), and bicarbonate. A **salt** is formed from a metal and a nonmetal. The most familiar salt is sodium chloride, or common table salt.

In bones and teeth, minerals are found in the form of salts (mainly as calcium and phosphates). In solution, salts dissolve. They are found in the bodily fluids as Na^+ (sodium), K^+ (potassium), Ca^{++} (calcium), Cl^- (chloride), and $H_2PO_4^{-2}$ (phosphate).

$$NaCl + H_2O \rightarrow Na^+ + Cl^-$$

Salt dissolves in water

In cancer patients mineral deficiencies can result from several factors:

- Decreased mineral intake from loss of appetite or the poor selection of foods
- Decreased absorption as the result of radiation-damaged

villi, bowel inflammation, or not enough pancreatic enzymes

- Decreased utilization of minerals due to drug interactions or too little energy from food
- Increased losses of minerals due to diarrhea, vomiting, or drug therapy
- Increased requirement due to tumor growth

The Macro Minerals

There are seven macro minerals: calcium, phosphorus, magnesium, sulfur, sodium, potassium, and chloride.

Calcium and Phosphorus

Calcium and phosphorus are very closely related to each other, so we will discuss them together. Calcium is the most abundant mineral in the body, comprising 39 percent of the minerals present in the body. Of this calcium, 99 percent is stored in the bones, teeth, and hard tissues. The remaining 1 percent is found in the tissues and extracellular fluid, where it is very active metabolically.

Phosphorus is the second most abundant mineral. Eighty percent of it is found in the bones and teeth. The remaining 20 percent is distributed to every cell of the body and extracellular fluid, where it is involved in numerous chemical reactions.

In bone, calcium and phosphorus are present as calcium carbonate and calcium phosphate. These two salts are arranged together in a crystal structure around a matrix of softer protein material. This structure is called **hydroxyapatite**. It provides strength and hardness to the bone.

Calcium is also needed for certain enzymes involved in energy production, for proper blood clotting, and muscle contraction. It affects transportation across cellular and subcellular membranes. It influences the release of neurotransmitters and the release and activation of enzymes. Calcium is required for nerve transmission and to regulate the heartbeat.

Phosphorus is the most active of the minerals. It is involved in almost every metabolic function of the body. In its most important function, phosphate acts as an energy currency. This energy is stored in a rechargeable battery known as **adenosine triphosphate (ATP)**. When energy is needed for a chemical reaction, an ATP molecule comes to the site from the mitochondria. The needed energy is stored in one of the phosphate-to-carbon bonds. The ATP molecule breaks the bond, and the energy is freed for the chemical reaction. What is left is **adenosine diphosphate (ADP)** and a free phosphate group. ADP molecules and free phosphate groups wander back to the mitochondria, where they are recharged with the energy released from burning glucose.

Several factors increase the body's absorption of calcium and phosphate:

- Acidity of the gastric juice—The hydrochloric acid present in the stomach lowers the pH (increases the acidity) of the chyme (undigested food) in the digestive tract to a level more favorable to calcium and phosphate absorption.
- Fat intake—When fat is present in the digestive tract, it slows the movement of chyme, giving more time for mineral absorption.
- Protein intake—A high intake of protein favors a higher absorption of calcium and phosphorus.
- Vitamin D—The active form of vitamin D stimulates intestinal absorption.
- State of need—When calcium levels are low, the body will absorb it more efficiently. When more calcium is needed for growth, it is better absorbed. As the body ages, the absorption decreases.

Phosphorus is so widely distributed in the food supply that it is almost impossible not to get enough. A much bigger problem is the large amounts of phosphorus taken in as phosphates

(PO$_4$) in prepared foods and sodas. Too many phosphates causes an imbalance, leading to a loss of calcium through the urine. The phosphorus (P) in unrefined foods poses no threat.

Sources of calcium include fortified soymilk, fortified orange juice, nonfat dairy products, tofu, corn tortillas, collard and turnip greens, kale, and broccoli.

Magnesium

Magnesium is the atom responsible for the green color of chlorophyll. Therefore, if a vegetable is green, it is a source of magnesium.

Magnesium and calcium have similar functions and may oppose each other. In normal muscle contraction, calcium acts as stimulator and magnesium as relaxer. The presence of calcium, fat, alcohol, phosphate, and phytates decrease magnesium absorption. As dietary calcium is decreased, magnesium absorption is increased. The kidneys regulate magnesium excretion. When the level of magnesium intake is low, the kidneys reabsorb most of the magnesium so that very little is lost.

A deficiency in magnesium can be caused by not enough intake, persistent vomiting (the gastric juice is relatively high in magnesium that is normally totally reabsorbed), or rapid transport of food through the digestive tract. Both alcohol and diuretics increase the loss of magnesium through the urine.

Sources of magnesium include nuts, brewer's yeast, soybeans, dried apricots, collard greens, and whole-grain cereals.

Sulfur

Sulfur is present in every cell of the body. The highest concentrations are in the hair, skin, and nails.

It has several functions:

- Sulfur is a part of three vitamins: thiamine, pantothenic acid, and biotin.

- Sulfur compounds act as detoxifying agents by combining with toxic substances, converting them into harmless ones, which are then excreted.
- It is involved in the formation of blood clots and in the transfer of energy.

Sulfur is obtained primarily through the sulfur-containing amino acids methionine and cysteine. Any excess of organic sulfur is excreted in the urine.

Electrolytes

Sodium, potassium, and chloride are known collectively as the electrolytes. Electrolytes carry the electrical currents for all the cells of the body. There must be a perfect balance of electrolytes for proper muscle movement, brain activity, and heart functions. Vomiting and diarrhea can seriously deplete electrolytes and in rare cases cause life-threatening complications.

Do not attempt to supplement electrolytes with sports drinks. These are designed for water loss due to vigorous exercise. Fruit and vegetable juices are frequently recommended as electrolyte replacements, but they are too concentrated and often too sweet. Sugary drinks may increase vomiting. You can purchase prepared electrolyte replacement solutions in the drugstore or the baby food section of your grocery store.

The Trace Minerals

The trace minerals include iron, zinc, copper, selenium, chromium, iodine, manganese, cobalt, arsenic, boron, molybdenum, nickel, silicon, vanadium, cadmium, lead, lithium, bromine, fluorine, and tin.

The remaining trace minerals have only begun to be studied. It is known that they are needed in minute amounts, and some, such as lead and cadmium, may even be poisonous if taken in excess. In general the best sources of trace minerals are whole foods and in particular whole grains.

Iron

The red in the red blood cells comes from iron. As the active compound in hemoglobin, it is the carrier of oxygen from the lungs and to the tissues and the carrier of carbon dioxide from the tissues back to the lungs. Iron is the reason muscles are red. It is also the active part of myoglobin, the iron-containing compound that provides oxygen to muscle cells. It is an important part of many different enzymes.

The combination of foods eaten influences the amount of iron absorbed. The iron in cereal grains is bound to phytic acid, forming an insoluble iron-phytate complex. When a vitamin C source is eaten along with the grain, this complex is broken, freeing both the iron and the phytic acid (which is linked to decreased cancer risk as well). Iron losses occur

Iron-Rich Foods

FOOD	IRON CONTENT (MILLIGRAMS)
clams, canned, 3 ounces	12.8
sunflower seeds, kernels, ½ cup	4.9
oyster, cooked, 3 ounces	4.4
cashews, ½ cup	4.1
shrimp, boiled, 3½ ounces	3.1
lentils, cooked, ½ cup	3.1
potato, baked with skin, 1 medium	2.8
kidney beans, cooked, ½ cup	2.6
refried beans, cooked, ½ cup	2.2
prunes, dried, 10	2.1
trout, baked or broiled, 3 ounces	2.1
almonds, ½ cup	2.5
turkey, roasted, dark meat, 3 ounces	2.0
black beans, cooked, ½ cup	1.8
apricot halves, dried, ½ cup	1.7
artichoke, 1 whole	1.6
peas, cooked, ½ cup	1.6
raisins, ½ cup	1.5
chicken, roasted, dark meat, 3 ounces	1.1

from loss of blood due to menstruation or minute bleeding in the intestine. For example, each 500 milligrams of aspirin a person takes can cause the loss of up to one teaspoon of blood.

The following practices will help increase iron absorption:

- Eat a *small* amount (one or two tablespoons) of fish or skinless poultry with a meal.
- Cook in an iron pot. It can add substantial amounts of dietary iron, particularly when the food being cooked is acidic such as tomato sauce.
- Eat foods rich in malic, ascorbic, or citric acid.
- Avoid coffee, tea, and spinach with iron-rich meals. These foods contain compounds that decrease mineral absorption.

Zinc

The trace mineral zinc is vital for the metabolism of vitamin A and has important roles in many of the body's systems, including immune function and wound healing. Dietary zinc is necessary for the working of many metal-containing enzymes, stabilizes membranes, and is needed for growth.

In people with cancer, low levels of zinc can reduce the ability to taste. This can contribute to a lack of appetite during treatment. Low zinc levels can slow wound healing from surgery and tissue regrowth of radiation- and chemotherapy-damaged tissues. Insufficient zinc affects T cell and NK cell activity, thereby decreasing the ability of the immune system to defend itself.

Zinc is necessary for the proper use of insulin, the hormone that regulates blood sugar. This is important for people with cancer, because the disease alters blood sugar metabolism.

Whole grains are much better sources of zinc (and other minerals) than refined. Even though the zinc from refined grains is better absorbed than the zinc from whole grains, the whole grain contains more zinc to begin with.

Zinc supplements should be taken between meals separately

from other supplements to prevent them from competing for absorption.

Sources of zinc include nuts, whole grains, shellfish, split peas, lima beans, sardines, anchovies, haddock, turnips, potatoes, egg yolk, soy lecithin, almonds, walnuts, and garlic.

Copper

Copper plays an important but poorly understood role in iron metabolism. In fact, anemia was first described as a copper deficiency. Copper is necessary for the proper functioning of the immune system, and animal studies have linked copper deficiency with decreased activity of NK cells. It is a part of superoxide dismutase, an enzyme necessary for protection from free radicals.

How well copper is absorbed depends on what the meal contains. The high doses of vitamin C we recommend will decrease absorption of copper, so you must supplement extra copper at a different time. High amounts of fructose have the same effect. This is why we do not recommend fructose as a purified sweetener. The presence of zinc will also decrease absorption, due to the competition for absorption sites.

Copper can leach from copper water pipes and holding tanks, cooking pots, and eating utensils.

Sources of copper include shellfish and legumes.

Selenium

Animal studies indicate that selenium inhibits the formation of tumors and may slow their growth. It is also a cofactor of glutathione peroxidase, an enzyme that is an integral part of the body's defenses against free radicals. When zinc levels are low, antibody production and the activity of NK cells are decreased. There is also evidence that selenium may be directly toxic to tumors. Selenium works synergistically with vitamin E to protect the lipids in cell membranes.

The optimal supplementation level is 200 micrograms per

day. Never let the total amount of zinc in all your supplements exceed 800 micrograms; it could be toxic.

Sources of selenium include swordfish and Brazil nuts (the two most concentrated sources), salmon, tuna, lobster, shrimp, oysters, haddock, sunflower seeds, barley, brown rice, and red Swiss chard.

Chromium
Chromium is part of glucose tolerance factor, which works with insulin to see that it is absorbed and utilized by the cells. Cancer cells alter carbohydrate metabolism, causing high blood glucose levels. Chromium works to stabilize glucose levels in the blood, leaving less circulating fuel for the tumor.

Sources of chromium include whole grains and high-chromium brewer's yeast.

Summary
Mineral intake is difficult to measure. The total amount of any given mineral, calculated by adding the contribution of each component of the diet, does not accurately reflect how much of that mineral is actually going to be absorbed from a meal. Mineral absorption and utilization depend not only on how much of a mineral is present in the meal, but on the other foods present in the stomach, the acidity in the stomach, the bioavailability of the mineral, mineral interactions, time of stay in the digestive tract, mineral stores in the body, and mineral needs. Mineral balance is also affected by how much is stored in the body and how much is excreted.

12

Phytochemicals and Cancer

$\mathcal{P}$hytochemicals come in such a wide variety of forms and functions that they are difficult to classify. This chapter will focus only on those properties that can aid you in your treatment plan. We will look at what phytochemicals are, where they come from, and how they support the immune system, increase enzyme levels, and prevent metastasis.

For many years a food's nutritional value was determined by its vitamin, mineral, and energy content. The old adage of an apple a day was deemed a myth, for the lowly apple had little of these to offer. It lacked the vitamin C found in citrus fruits, the calcium found in leafy greens, and the complex carbohydrates found in potatoes. In short, it was a nutritional bust. Down to the bottom of the vegetable pile for the once proud apple.

Then fiber was "discovered." America was constipated, and this was the cure. Dubbed "nature's broom," roughage was judged necessary to keep the colon clean and tidy. The apple advanced one notch to a laxative by virtue of its fiber.

Today the new kid on the nutrition block is the phytochemical (*phyto* = plant). Also called nutraceuticals and anutrients, **phytochemicals** are naturally occurring plant compounds that the human body has learned to use in novel ways. They are not related chemically to each other and have no deficiency symptoms. In fact, most of them have yet to be discovered. Chemicals such as polyphenols that kill viruses, glutathione that quenches free radicals, and pectin, which reduces cholesterol, suddenly became the "in" topic. And, you guessed it, all of these can be found in the apple. Back to the top of the heap again!

You can often tell how good a source of phytochemicals a food is by your eyes and nose. Pigments have antioxidant properties, with orange beta-carotene being the most familiar. Strong odors are often associated with phytochemicals such as the sulfur-containing compounds that give cabbage and the other cruciferous vegetables their distinctive aroma. Other phytochemicals are less obvious. But nature has not wasted any part of a plant. We may not understand why or how phytochemicals work, but it is an undeniable fact that whole foods promote health and prevent disease.

Let's begin with some of the larger phytochemical families.

Carotenoids

The carotenoids are a huge family of over 600 yellow to red pigments, of which beta-carotene is the most famous. Each carotenoid is unique, so different carotenoids are preferred by different organs. The cells in your liver, heart, thyroid gland, kidneys, and pancreas prefer beta-carotene and lycopene equally, while the cells of the adrenal glands and testes mainly prefer just lycopene. Zeaxanthin and beta-carotene are favorites in the ovaries, and in the macula of the eye lutein and zeaxanthin predominate.

Beta-carotene is the object of most research and has been

Carotenoid Food Groups

ALPHA- AND BETA-CAROTENE	BETA-CRYPTOXANTHIN	ZEAXANTHIN
carrots	oranges	peaches
sweet potatoes	grapefruit	corn
pumpkin	lemons	**LUTEIN AND BETA-CAROTENE**
winter squash	tangerines	deep green leafy vegetables
yams	**LYCOPENE**	**ASTAXANTHIN**
GAMMA-CAROTENE	tomatoes	salmon
tomatoes	watermelon	

shown to have antitumor effects by causing regression and redifferentiation of established cancers. However alpha-carotene can be up to ten times more effective in this manner. See Chapter 5 on the immune system for more information on these pigments.

How to Supplement Beta-Carotene

Do not take large amounts of beta-carotene in purified form. In amounts over 20,000 IU, pure beta carotene has been shown to depress the blood-circulating levels of other, more important carotenoids. This may be due to competition for absorption.

Do take a supplement that contains a mixture of naturally occurring carotenoids. This includes but is not limited to beta- and alpha-carotene, lutein, cryptoxanthin, and lycopene.

An IU (international unit of activity) refers to the amount of vitamin A the body can make from the dose. However, most xanthophylls and lycopene do not have provitamin A activity and therefore have no IU activity. Xanthophylls and lycopene should be listed in milligrams, not in international units.

Check the color of the supplement. It should be orange to red. If not, it may contain little or no carotenoids. Or the supplement may be old and the pigments oxidized. The breakdown products of most carotenoids are colorless.

The Flavonoids

The flavonoid group of compounds was originally referred to as "vitamin P." The P stood for "permeability factor" (and for paprika, the source), since an extract of Hungarian peppers enhanced vitamin C's ability to repair the permeability of blood vessels found in scurvy. Today we know these citrus flavonoids are only one of many different types of flavonoids. Flavonoids are commonly referred to as bioflavonoids— meaning flavonoids with biologic activity.

Flavonoids, like the carotenes, are pigments. They produce a wide variety of colors in fruits and vegetables, from the colorless flavonones in citrus fruit to the red and blue anthocyanins in berries, and are usually concentrated in the peel, skin, or outer layer of the plant. Tea and wine are also sources of bioflavonoids. They appear to work synergistically with vitamin C and work to stimulate the detoxification of drugs by the liver enzymes.

Bioflavonoids important to cancer patients include the following:

- Quercetin is the most commonly occurring flavonoid. It blocks the manufacture of the prostaglandin E2 series, which can depress the immune system, and may be directly toxic to cancer cells.
- Rutin, a flavonoid found in buckwheat, may also be toxic to cancer cells. It is an important antioxidant that strengthens the capillaries.
- Aglycone, kaempferol, and myricetin are flavonoids found in green and black tea. They are responsible for the potent cancer-fighting and antioxidant properties of Japanese green tea.

Cruciferous Vegetables

The National Cancer Institute has linked the cruciferous vegetables to a reduced risk of colon cancer and protective effects against cancer of the lung, esophagus, larynx, rectum, colon, lung, stomach, prostate, and bladder. Cruciferous vegetables contain such potential cancer-preventing or cancer-inhibiting substances as aromatic isothiocyanates (benzyl isothiocyanate, phenethyl isothiocyanate), glucosinolates (glucobrassin, glucotropaeolin), flavones, indoles, and phenols. Some of these phytochemicals stop carcinogens before they have a chance to alter DNA structure. Others slow the development or spread of cancerous cells or stimulate the release of anticancer enzymes. Indoles increase the detoxification of estrogen, reducing that hormone's chance of enhancing cancer growth in hormone-sensitive cells.

These vegetables also contain the antioxidant vitamins A,

C, and E, which clean up cancer-promoting free radicals, and are good sources of soluble and insoluble fiber.

Seasonings

Garlic is a natural antibiotic that will help stave off bacterial and viral infections. Eating garlic after cancer treatments when immune functioning is low will increase protection from infections. Garlic contains **organosulfur compounds** (siallyl sulfide, diallyl disulfide, allyl mercaptan, allyl methyl disulfide) that block carcinogenic activation, increase carcinogenic detoxification, and block tumor growth. Other members of the allium family with similar properties include onions, leeks, and shallots. Since garlic is a potent antibiotic, it should never be taken or eaten in megadoses.

Shiitake, maitake, and reishi mushrooms contain lenitan, a biological response modifier that increases immune system response to cancer cells. Enjoy the mushrooms or supplements that are available.

Other seasonings with medicinal effects are the following:

* Rosemary contains four different antioxidants that help increase immune function.
* Ginger in fresh or powdered form is as effective as popular antinausea drugs for curbing motion sickness. Before chemotherapy starts, try it to reduce nausea.
* Peppermint stimulates bile flow and the appetite and aids digestion.
* Nutmeg can reduce peristalsis of the gastrointestinal tract during diarrhea.

Soy Products

The consumption of soy products by people with cancer has been dubbed the "tofu treatment." As silly as it sounds, the tofu treatment really works. One cup of soybeans contains twenty-eight grams of protein (half the RDA), fiber, zinc, B vitamins, half a day's supply of iron, and loads of highly absorbable calcium. Just on the basis of their vitamin and mineral content, soyfoods are of therapeutic value. What is special about soyfoods, however, is the types of phytochemicals present in them.

Soy products appear to inhibit breast cancer by decreasing the level of circulating estrogen, thereby blocking the cancer-promoting action of estrogen. One serving a day of soy may decrease the risk of developing a number of cancers by nearly 40 percent. Soy also has a cholesterol-lowering effect. Some of the phytochemicals found in soy include the following:

- Phytoesterols help protect against heart disease and are effective against skin cancer.
- Saponins are antioxidants and play a role in cancer prevention.
- Genistein, an isoflavone found in soy products, is protective against colon, breast, lung, prostate, and skin cancer and leukemia.
- Daidzein, another isoflavone, has slowed the growth of breast cancer cells in vivo.
- Protease inhibitors appear to inhibit or prevent cancer growth.

Summary

One of the reasons a whole-food diet is so healthful is that it provides many phytochemicals. These substances can have a profound effect on the immune system. The best way to get these compounds is through eating a varied diet. Food pills, juice pills, and the like are only pale imitations of real foods.

Part II

Friendly Fire:
The Nutritional
Side Effects
of Treatment

*U*nlike my husband, who never worries and has no nerve endings to speak of, I was and still am, a weenie, a wimp, a wuss. My body does not recognize the existence of small pains: either something does not hurt at all, or it hurts terribly—usually the latter. New experiences are not something I treasure or seek voluntarily. Needles, doctors, and hospitals send my blood pressure plummeting. Needless to say, the stage was neatly set for one of the worst experiences of my life.

But it didn't happen that way. I got through it. Cancer treatment was not fun, and I certainly have no desire to repeat the experience, but I would not let it get the better of me. I took control of what I could and let go of what I couldn't. I read, I researched, I visualized, and I prayed.

As the start of therapy drew near, I was petrified. I had heard all of the usual horror stories; so have you, I'm sure. But the chemotherapy was not really that bad, and the surgery was uncomfortable but not painful. Sixteen years later it makes a terrific story, almost as good as my childbirth horrors.

The first two courses of chemotherapy were the worst. The methotrexate caused a loss of hair, very painful sores on my tongue, a sore throat, pustules on my forehead, nausea, fatigue, and headaches. But I got myself a wig, stuffed my mouth with Xylocaine-saturated cotton, and taught my Irish dance classes by holding up signs. I slicked my hair over the pustules and danced in a show myself that St. Patrick's Day. The next two courses seemed easier to me but were actually harder on my body. The actinomycin seemed only to cause fatigue, but both courses of it ended early because of liver damage. And I still continued to teach dancing while trying to dodge the four-year-old twins, who always attempted to yank off my wig. While you may not feel like dancing a jig during your treatment, it does help to stay on your regular routine as much as possible.

You are probably familiar with the old axiom, "You are what you eat." But the opposite is also true: "You eat what you are." When you are feeling poorly from cancer treatments or the cancer itself, your diet also is apt to be poor. When I was in treatment, I had a very active toddler, and getting my husband and son fed often took up most of my energy. I put my needs last.

This has to change. If you have young children, discuss sharing cooking responsibilities with your spouse. Older children and teens can be pressed into service to help feed younger ones. The job of the digestive system is to take in nutrients that the immune system needs, but your main job now is getting nutritious food into your stomach.

Maureen Keane

13

....

Food Preparation

$\mathcal{H}$ow you prepare your food is almost as important as how you choose your food. It does your body no good to take a piece of EPA-rich salmon and deep-fry it into nuggets of saturated fat. Likewise, boiling fresh organic vegetables in water until their bodies are limp shadows of their former nutrient-rich selves makes no sense. This chapter will give some preparation tips to make eating a pleasure while you are in treatment. If you are already in treatment and are short on energy or patience, give this work to your spouse, friends, and family. It will give them a constructive way to show their concern.

Juicing

Juicing is the victim of black-or-white reasoning. Supporters believe the "juice pushers" on the TV infomercials and consider fresh juices a cure for everything. Critics dismiss the whole idea as another silly fad. The truth, as always, lies somewhere in between.

Juice extractors work by splitting open the cell wall of the plant and separating the cytoplasm and other liquid components from the cell walls and other fibrous parts. The liquid portion, or juice, contains the contents of the plastids and vacuoles, any vitamin, mineral, flavor components, and some of the pectins that were in the cytoplasm. The solid portion, or pulp, contains the cellulose, lignin, and remaining pectins found in the cell walls. Since juices by definition lack fiber, they should never be used to replace the five fruits and vegetables a day your body needs.

Juices have been criticized because they lack fiber, but their therapeutic value lies in just this quality. The average person would have difficulty eating a pound of carrots, but this same amount juiced becomes a quickly consumed eight ounces. A juicer will allow you to increase your consumption of fruits and vegetables at a time when you may not feel like eating due to mouth sores, sore throat, difficulty in chewing and swallowing, early satiety, lack of appetite, or just plain dislike of vegetables in general. It is the only way to get fruits and vegetables into you when on a low-fiber diet.

As handy as food supplements are, they cannot replace whole foods. Consider for example, beta-carotene supplements. We are told that in large doses beta-carotene is nontoxic, and it is. The more beta-carotene consumed, the higher are the blood levels of beta-carotene. But high beta-carotene levels are also associated with a decrease in blood levels of the other carotenes, some of which are more powerful antioxidants than beta-carotene. Recent studies indicate that beta-carotene may compete for absorption with the other carotenes.

Juice, unlike purified supplements, contains all of the carotenes present in the juiced food. So while juice is not a whole food, it is a wholesome food, and quite a few steps closer to whole than food supplements. Just be sure not to overdo it. I have talked to people who were drinking a gallon or two a day and to others who were consuming no foods, only juices. Please do not stress your body this way. Without adequate protein, your body will not be able to fight the cancer. One or two glasses of fresh vegetable juice is all you need.

Evaluate a juicer as you would any electrical appliance. The juice that is produced is the same, regardless of the type of machine. What differs between machines is the power of the motor and the ease of cleaning. We recommend a pulp ejector type, since they are the easiest to clean. Juice extractors can be found in any department store and some health food stores.

Pressure-Cooking

When you are tired or not feeling well from therapy, who wants to stand over a hot stove and cook? Pull up a chair and let a pressure cooker do the work for you.

The advantages of today's safety-conscious pressure cookers are many:

- Pressure cookers prepare foods faster than any other cooking method, including the microwave. They make fast food healthy food. Whole grains such as brown rice cook in less than fifteen minutes.
- Food comes out moist, tender, and easy to swallow—important attributes when the mouth is dry or sore.
- The cooker seals in flavors and nutrients. Vegetables not only look great, but all of their flavors are retained, not lost to the air.
- Cooking odors are sealed into the pot. Food odor will not linger in the air for hours after, killing your appetite.
- By using the metal trivet in the cooker, you can cook foods in the serving dish, making cleanup a snap. This is a wonderful way to cook only one serving.

Skip the smaller models and buy one with a capacity of at least six quarts. This will enable you to pressure-steam foods in their serving dishes or let you cook a whole meal at once. Pressure cookers are currently enjoying a revival. They can be found in most department stores and discount houses.

Food Steaming

Food steamers make grain and vegetable cooking simply goof proof. They are not as fast as pressure cookers, but they do not need to be watched. Just add the food and come back when the timer goes off. Steamers are particularly suited for delicate vegetables such as leafy greens. Small grains like quinoa or millet that can get gummy when cooked in a saucepan come out separate, fluffy, and much more appetizing in a steamer.

Food steamers come in many shapes and sizes. We suggest

you buy a plastic food steamer rather than a metal rice cooker. The food steamers are much easier to clean and more versatile.

Here's a summary of the benefits:

- You can't burn the pan with the steamer because it will automatically turn itself off when the water runs out.
- Steaming is one of the easiest ways to cook the whole grains necessary for colon health. Cook a week's worth of your favorite grain, and store it in the refrigerator. For a quick meal add a few tablespoons of the cooked grain to the steamer with some chopped leafy greens. Sprinkle with a marinade and reheat.
- Water-soluble flavors and vitamins are not lost to boiling water. Foods taste better and are better for you.
- Steamed foods are moist and tender. They do not hurt sore gum and mouth tissues and are easy to swallow when the throat is dry.
- Food steamers allow you to cook food in the serving bowl, making cleanup quick. Most plastic parts just require a simple wipe to clean.

As with the pressure cookers, larger is better. Buy one with a built-in timer so you will not have to remember when to turn it off. Food steamers are inexpensive and available everywhere.

14

Guidelines for Oral Health

You depend on your teeth and gums to prepare the food you eat for digestion. When they are diseased or painful, good nutrition becomes difficult. Since many cancer treatments will cause soreness or pain to the tissues of the mouth, gums, and throat, these structures must be in good condition to start with. Before starting your cancer treatment program, start a program of oral health to protect your mouth from developing infections that can undermine your treatment and the ability of your body to heal.

Before Treatment Begins

See your dentist for a pretreatment evaluation. If you have any difficulty eating with your teeth, now is the time to have cavities filled and other dental work done.

Inform your dentist about your health problems. Extraction and other oral surgeries must be done at least a month in advance to give oral tissues time to heal. Once cancer therapy begins, healing and tissue regeneration will stop. This can result in permanent dental problems.

Have your teeth cleaned. A clean mouth will give bacteria and fungi no place to hide and feed.

If you wear dentures, make sure that they fit properly without causing any irritations.

During Treatment

Once treatment begins, follow a strict dental health regime at home:

- Brush your teeth gently, three times a day, with a soft-bristle toothbrush. Use a nonabrasive fluoride toothpaste.

- Floss teeth every day to remove trapped food and tartar.
- If your gums become too sore to brush, clean around gums with a soft cloth. Use a nonirritating toothpaste. A paste of baking soda and water makes a gentle but refreshing cleaner.
- Avoid mouthwashes that contain alcohol. They can irritate tissues.
- Rinse your mouth with water after drinking or eating sweet foods or juices.
- Mouth irritations and sores can be relieved by the topical application of vitamin E or tea tree oil.
- Make sure your toothbrush does not become a breeding place for germs. Replace it often, and always rinse it well and leave to air dry before putting it away.

15

Nausea and Vomiting

One of the most common side effects of cancer treatment is gastrointestinal upset. This chapter shows how nutrition therapy can help you cope.

Most of the time gastrointestinal tract upset is minor and does not last long. In many cases, the nausea and vomiting disappear when the treatment is stopped. In severe or prolonged cases, it is necessary to take an antiemetic drug so that the body is able to get the nutrients it needs. Although some people may balk at taking yet another drug, good nutrition at this point is more important.

Vomiting is how the body gets rid of food that should not be in the stomach. It is stimulated by sensory receptors in the wall of the stomach, including stretch receptors that indicate when the stomach is too full and chemoreceptors that detect

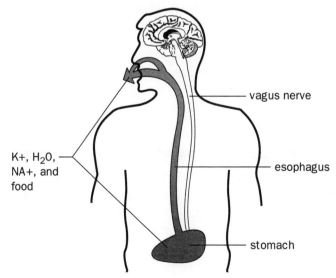

Vomiting input from sensors

possible toxins and poisons. The emetic center in the brain responds to these signals as well as to the presence of possible toxic substances in the blood by causing a wave of reverse peristalsis expelling the contents.

While vomiting is unpleasant and even painful when coupled with a raw throat and mouth sores, it is only dangerous when it is severe or prolonged. The main danger is loss of fluids and electrolytes from the body, causing dehydration, weight loss, and an electrolyte imbalance. In severe cases intravenous fluids may be needed to reverse the imbalances.

Words to Know

Nausea—Upset stomach.
Anticipatory Nausea—An upset stomach before treatment caused by the thought of treatment or even the sight of the hospital or clinic where treatment is given.
Emesis—Vomiting.
Emetic center—The area of the brain that controls vomiting.
Antiemetics—Drugs that reduce nausea and vomiting.
Emetogenic potential—The ability of a drug to cause nausea and vomiting. Drugs such as cisplatin, dacarbazine, and mechlorethamine have a high emetogenic potential, since they cause nausea and vomiting in over 90 percent of patients.
Food Aversions—A phenomenon where foods eaten close to the time of a nausea-causing treatment become linked in the brain with the symptoms caused by a treatment. Aromatic foods are at greatest risk for this.

Learned food aversions are also possible. Immediately after my first chemotherapy treatment, I went to a luncheon where freshly grated horseradish was served with corned beef. I was nauseated at the time, and the back of my hand hurt from the IV. For ten years, every time I smelled horseradish or corned beef, I would get nauseated and the back of my hand would hurt.

This reaction is not at all uncommon. To prevent it from

destroying the enjoyment of your favorite foods, do not eat them immediately before or after treatments. Not all of these suggestions will work for every person. Sometimes the best thing to do is to listen to the wisdom of your body and eat whatever nutritious food you can tolerate or enjoy.

Causes of Nausea

- *Chemotherapy*—The most common side effect from chemotherapy is nausea and vomiting. Chemotherapy causes nausea by acting on both the brain and stomach. The emetic center in the brain that controls vomiting may be stimulated by the drugs. Some drugs work on the stomach itself, causing local irritation that results in upset.
- *Stress*—The stress from fear, pain, or phobias (e.g., of needles, hospitals, blood) is often overlooked as a cause of stomach upset. For some of us, the first sign of stress is an upset stomach.
- *Radiation*—Radiation of the spine and skull for central nervous system tumors often causes nausea. Radiation treatment to the gastrointestinal tract will also cause upset soon after administration, as can total body irradiation conditioning for bone marrow transplant.

Solutions

Plan ahead. Get ready to combat the problem with these tactics:

- Ask your physician about the emetic potential of your treatment plan and the advisability of an antiemetic drug. The drug must be taken before treatment begins if it is to be effective.
- If stress first manifests itself in your stomach or if you are phobic of hospitals, needles, blood, or IVs, be prepared for stress-induced nausea.

- Arrange for someone else to prepare your food. If that is not possible, prepare foods ahead of time. Pack foods into single-serving bags that are ready to eat when you are.
- A few hours before treatment, place an acupressure band around your wrist. These bands stimulate the acupressure point that relieves nausea. They are available in most drugstores and pharmacies.

Before and During Treatment:
- If you react to stress with stomach butterflies, remember to breathe from your abdomen deeply and slowly. It's amazing how many people forget to breathe during stressful situations.
- Do not eat for two hours before or after chemotherapy treatment. The drugs can stimulate the stomach and emetic center in the brain to produce nausea.
- Avoid eating highly flavored or aromatic foods the day of treatment. When eaten again, they can cause a "nausea flashback."

To Prevent Nausea After Treatment
- Eat small, frequent meals rather than three large ones, and do not drink large amounts of liquids with the meals. Too much food or liquid can overexpand the stomach, activating the stretch receptors and stimulating the emetic center. For the same reason, do not drink carbonated or fizzy beverages.
- Position is important. Sit up to eat and do not lie down immediately after. A prone position can cause the food to back up into the esophagus.
- Make mealtimes calm and relaxing. Read or watch TV while eating. Rest and relax (in a sitting position) after eating. Avoid arguments or confrontations during mealtimes.

- Avoid cooking odors. Strong food aromas can be reduced by using a pressure cooker to prepare family meals. Odor neutralizers are handy to keep around. These products remove smells instead of masking them with a perfumy odor. They come in spray bottles and are often marketed as pet odor removers.
- Heavy perfumes and smoke odors can also provoke nausea. Buy cleaning products and personal care items that are marked as unscented or fragrance free. (The perfumy odor of fabric softener sheets in the clothes dryer used to make me nauseous.)
- Do not eat greasy or high-fat foods. Fat causes food to remain in the stomach longer, increasing the chance you may vomit. Avoid all deep-fried foods, meat, whole milk and cheeses, butter, oils, salad dressings, potato and corn chips, and nut butters, including peanut butter and tahini.
- Eat foods that are easy to digest, such as crackers, lightly salted pretzels, dry toast, and soft bread. Avoid raw or highly fibrous foods, and chew each mouthful thoroughly. Later in the day eat a low-fat, high-protein food such as skinless chicken breast, mild fish, or a legume soup.
- Avoid foods with strong odors or flavors such as onions, garlic, horseradish, cabbage, broccoli, cauliflower, brussels sprouts and other members of the cruciferous family, eggs, hot peppers, and any other highly spiced foods. Avoid any food that "repeats" on you.

To Relieve Nausea After Treatment
- Cold nonacid liquids often help to settle a stomach. This includes small sips of ice water, ice chips, iced herbal teas, iced tea, and small tastes of all-fruit sorbets.
- Clear or salty liquids are easy to keep down. Miso soup and broths are nutritious choices. Peppermint tea calms some stomachs.
- If you do not feel like eating, don't. Listen to your

stomach, and wait until the nausea passes.

- Ginger capsules will often help to relieve nausea but will not work once you have started to vomit.
- Place an ice pack on the back of your neck. Keep a supply of gel pacs in the freezer for quick use.
- Open some windows and let in fresh, cool air. Stuffy, stale, or smoky air will make nausea worse and increase the chance of vomiting.
- Keep your teeth and tongue clean, brushed, and flossed and your mouth rinsed. This will help keep bad flavors and odors from developing.

Severe Nausea

If the suggestions listed do not work, call your doctor or nurse. You may need IV hydration and electrolytes.

16

Dry Mouth and Difficulty Swallowing

$\mathcal{A}$ dry mouth makes chewing and swallowing difficult. Since saliva keeps the mouth clean, the dry mouth can also become a breeding ground for bacteria, which can promote tooth decay and cause infections. Good oral hygiene is necessary to prevent these when the immune system is depressed due to treatment.

Words to Know

Xerostomia—A decrease in saliva that causes the sensation of a dry mouth.
Dysphagia—Difficulty in swallowing.
Salivary glands—The glands that secrete saliva, including the large parotid, submaxillary, and sublingual glands.
Saliva—A mixture of secretions from the salivary and oral mucous glands that keeps the tissues of the mouth moist and lubricates food to facilitate swallowing.
Sialagogue—A drug or other agent that increases the flow of saliva.

Causes

- *Chemotherapy*—Some chemotherapeutic agents such as bleomycin and dactinomycin cause a temporary dryness of the mouth. Antinausea drugs may also have this effect.
- *Radiation*—Radiation to the neck or head may cause damage to the salivary glands. This may result in a decrease in the amount of saliva or in the quality of the saliva, making it thick or viscous.

- *Surgery*—Surgery to the head or neck that removes one or more of the salivary glands will reduce secretions according to the extent of the surgery.

Solutions

Before Meals

Tart tastes will stimulate salivary flow. Add a tablespoon of fresh or frozen lemon juice to a small glass of water. Drink it fifteen minutes before mealtime.

During Meals

- Eat smaller, more frequent meals instead of three large ones.
- Avoid dry or sticky foods such as crackers, bread, or nut butters.
- Take small sips of water as you chew. This makes the food easier to swallow.
- Do not try to chew large pieces of food. Cut food into bite-sized pieces that are easier to swallow.
- Eat moist foods such as casseroles, stews, soups, fruits, and liquids.
- Add extra sauces, gravies, and broth to foods.
- Add vinegar, pickles, or lemon juice to food to stimulate saliva.

Between Meals

- Keep a small water bottle with you and take frequent sips. My favorite is a slim plastic bottle with a pop-up top that held a "designer" water. The water was quickly gone but the bottle has lasted for months. Carry your bottle with you in your purse, coat, or briefcase. Keep water at your bedside for when you wake up with that "cottony" feeling.
- Suck on ice cubes or ice chips when they are available.

- A dry mouth is a haven for bacteria that can cause tooth decay or tissue infections. Keep teeth and tongue brushed and flossed and mouth tissues rinsed.
- Use a wetting agent for the mouth such as Salivart or Xero-lube. These can be purchased in drugstores and pharmacies.

17

....

Taste Alterations
and Anorexia

$\mathcal{W}$hen you find it difficult to eat for any reason, you must make every meal and every food count. Now is not the time to abandon good food habits. Although you can get needed calories from ice cream, there are ways to get sufficient calories without resorting to junk food.

The sensation of taste is a nutritional factor that is often overlooked. Taste changes are not life-threatening complications, but they can make good nutrition more difficult. Taste triggers the salivary glands necessary for proper chewing and swallowing and stimulates the flow of the gastric juices necessary for digestion. Loss of taste means a decrease in the pleasure found in eating, which can cause a decrease in appetite.

Taste Alterations

Stimulation of the taste buds results in four taste sensations: sweet, sour, bitter, and salty. The brain decides which type of taste by the ratio of degree of stimulation by these four sensations. All flavors are a combination of these taste bud sensations combined with sensations received by the olfactory (odor) receptors and the trigeminal nerves, which detect irritants such as hot peppers and mint. Since the taste buds are formed from fast-dividing epithelial tissue, they are particularly sensitive to cancer therapies.

Words to Know

Dysgeusia—A change in the sense of taste.
Hypogeusia—A decrease in the ability to taste.
Ageusia—Complete loss of the ability to taste.
Taste buds—Chemical receptors for the taste nerve fibers.
Mucositis—An inflammation of the mucous membranes, causing mouth sores.

Causes of Taste Alterations

- *Chemotherapy*—Taste alterations are associated with certain chemotherapeutic drugs. Cisplatin, 5-fluorouracil, dactinomycin, daunorubicin, and methotrexate are associated with taste alterations. Cyclophosphamide and vincristine may be tasted after injection. And any chemotherapeutic drug can cause a bitter or metallic taste in some people.
- *Radiation Therapy*—Radiation can injure or kill taste buds. Radiation to the head and neck causes a temporary loss of taste two to three weeks after treatment. It can last for several weeks. Total body irradiation in preparation for a bone marrow transplant also causes injury. The taste buds recover forty-five to sixty days after transplantation.
- *Surgery*—Surgical removal of parts of the mouth that perceive taste will cause a permanent loss of those taste receptors. Sweet and salty sensations are eliminated after removal of the tongue. Removal of palate results in the loss of most sour and bitter receptor sites.
- *Infection*—Oral infections causing inflammation of the mucous membranes (mucositis) may decrease taste sensations, since the taste receptor cells become inflamed.

Solutions

Use these pointers before and during treatment:

- Do not eat favorite foods before chemotherapy treatment. The changes in taste may cause an unpleasant asso-

ciation with the food. Snack on crackers or unsalted pretzels instead.
- If chemotherapy causes a bad taste in your mouth, suck on a lemon drop or peppermint candy during treatment.

After treatment or surgery, follow these guidelines:
- If you develop a low threshold for bitter tastes, avoid beef (yet another reason!). Substitute skinless white poultry, mild-tasting fish, soyfoods, nut butters, and legumes for a protein source.
- Depending on tolerance, either add or decrease salt in food.
- Use herbs, spices, flavor extracts, and marinades to increase the flavor of food. If the tissues of the mouth are inflamed, avoid any hot spices that may irritate sore membranes.
- Foods that are cold or at room temperature may be more palatable than hot ones.
- Appeal to the other senses to make up for the lack of taste. The smell of highly aromatic foods such as garlic and onions may make up for a lack of taste buds. Use a variety of colored vegetables to add eye appeal and a variety of textures to add mouth appeal to your meals.
- Unpleasant food odors may be confused with unpleasant tastes. See the section on nausea for tips on how to avoid them.
- Use plastic eating utensils instead of metallic ones.
- Drink filtered water. Carafe-type water purifiers are inexpensive and greatly reduce the chemical flavors and odors common in tap water.
- A zinc supplement may increase taste sensitivity. Ask your physician.
- Keep your mouth, tongue, and teeth clean and well rinsed to wash away bad tastes.

Words to Know

Anorexia—Loss of appetite or the desire to eat.
Cachexia—Loss of weight, fat, and muscle mass in patients who are eating adequate calories.
Satiety—The feeling of being full after a meal.
Early satiety—The feeling of fullness and loss of appetite after a small amount of food.
Bloating—Feeling of fullness.

Anorexia

Do not confuse the anorexia some cancer patients experience with anorexia nervosa, an eating disorder unrelated to cancer. Rather, early satiety may kill the appetite, making proper nutrition difficult to achieve. Loss of appetite results in weight loss, malnutrition, and decreased immunity to infections.

Causes of Anorexia

Anorexia does not have a single cause. It is the result of a number of factors:

- *Toxic effects of therapy*—Side effects of treatment such as nausea, sore mouth and throat, stomach cramps, and taste changes can all decrease the desire to eat.
- *Localized effects of the tumor*—Tumors in the gastrointestinal tract causing blockages can decrease appetite. Some tumors produce chemicals that affect the endocrine system, resulting in early satiety.
- *Surgery*—Surgical removal of any part of the gastrointestinal tract can decrease the ability and desire to eat.

Solutions

The following solutions apply to meal planning:

- Appetite is usually the greatest first thing in the morning, so plan to have the largest meal of the day for breakfast.
- Plan your meals and go shopping for the food yourself, if you are able.

- Eat six small meals a day instead of three large ones. Or take small bites of nutrient-dense foods every hour or so.
- Eat whenever you are hungry. Do not wait for mealtime.
- Keep cooking odors to a minimum.

When you eat, follow these hints:
- Liquid meals are often more appealing than solid ones. Drink fresh vegetable and fruit juices instead of whole vegetables and fruits, and drink soymilk rather than eat soybeans. Blenderize soft fruits such as bananas, and add them to protein shakes.
- Do not drink liquids with meals. Eat the most nutrient-dense foods in the meal first.
- Avoid low-calorie, low-protein foods and beverages such as tea, coffee, or soda pop. Beverages with a high percentage of water will kill your appetite and fill you up without providing calories or protein.
- Avoid raw vegetables. Puree steamed veggies and mix them with high-calorie foods.
- Add olive oil, canola oil, or high oleic safflower oil to foods to increase the fat content.

The following ideas may help you improve a decreased appetite:
- Canned food supplements, which can be purchased at the drugstore, are a handy source of balanced nutrition in a pinch.
- Light exercise may stimulate the appetite. Ask your doctor about taking light walks before meals.
- Create a relaxed eating atmosphere. Try enhancing the meal surroundings to make mealtime more appealing. Try candlelight, soft music, or a colorful table setting.
- Very sweet or tart foods may stimulate saliva. Suck on lemon wedges or try lemonade.

18

Oral and Esophageal Mucositis

*M*ucositis begins with the tissues feeling dry and looking red. The mouth and throat are sore. This is followed by swelling, ulcerations, and, in some severe cases, bleeding. This inflammation is painful and limits food intake and enjoyment. Talking becomes difficult, and often a headache accompanies the mouth pain. Because of the open sores, there is a chance for infection.

Words to Know

Mucositis—An inflammation of the mucous membrane lining of the mouth and esophagus.
Stomatitis—An inflammation of the oral cavity.
Ulcer—An inflamed, open sore on the mucous membranes.
Esophagitis—An inflammation of the lining of the esophagus.
Dysphagia—Difficulty swallowing.

Causes of Mucositis

- *Chemotherapy*—Prevents the division of the rapidly dividing mucous membrane cells of the tongue, cheek, lips, gums, and palate, as well as the floor of the mouth and esophagus. When the top layers of cells are shed, they are not replaced. This causes inflammation as early as three days after treatment, which can progress into ulcerations after a week. Among the chemotherapeutic drugs that cause the most severe mucositis are dactinomycin, plicamycin, methotrexate, and 5-fluorouracil.

- *Radiation*—Radiotherapy to the head and neck can cause damage to the mucous membranes of the mouth and throat. Inflammation begins about two weeks after therapy and starts to heal two weeks after the treatment ends. Radiation therapy to the thorax can cause inflammation to the esophagus and difficulty in swallowing.
- *Total Body Irradiation*—The preparation for bone marrow transplant is also a major cause of inflammation and ulcerations in the mouth and esophagus. This can develop as soon as four days after preparative chemotherapy and heals with marrow engraftment and the return of neutrophils.

Solutions

For Meals

- Eat soft, nonirritating foods such as nonfat yogurt, oatmeal, brown rice farina, quinoa and other soft, well-cooked whole grains, pureed vegetables, and mashed potatoes and yams.
- Serve foods lukewarm or cold, never hot to avoid burning already irritated tissue.
- Vegetable soups are easy on sore throats. If the pain is very severe, the soup can be processed in a blender to liquefy solids.
- Avoid acidic, tart, or spicy foods such as citrus and tomato juices and fruits, vinegar-based salad dressings and condiments, hot peppers, curry, chili, and pepper-containing condiments and seasonings. Do not drink alcohol.
- Avoid dry, rough foods such as granola and toast.
- Drink your raw vegetables by making a glass or two of fresh juice from nonacid vegetables such as carrot, celery, and apple.
- If sores are confined to the tongue, use a straw to bypass them.

For severe dysphagia and pain in swallowing, you may need to follow a liquid diet.

To Heal and Soothe Tissues

- Bite open a 400 IU capsule of vitamin E and swish it around your mouth before swallowing.
- Follow the recommendations for vitamin C supplementation. It will help with tissue healing.
- Apply tea tree oil directly to the sores. Tea tree oil (from the tree that produces tea leaves) acts as a topical antibiotic.
- Sucking on ice chips can soothe a sore throat and help numb mouth sores.
- Keep your mouth very clean. Even though it may hurt to brush your teeth, a neglected mouth is a breeding ground for bacteria that can enter your body though the sores.
- If pain is severe enough to prevent you from eating, call your doctor or nurse. Your doctor can prescribe a local anesthetic to numb ulcers and sore spots so that you can eat.

19

Constipation and Diarrhea

*T*wo colon-related problems that may affect people undergoing treatment for cancer are constipation and diarrhea. Fortunately, nutrition therapy offers remedies for both conditions.

Digestion takes place in the **alimentary canal**: a thirty-foot tube that runs through the center of your body. The purpose of the digestive system is not only digestion, but absorption of what is digested, storage of what is not, and excretion of waste products and undigested food. Food moves through the alimentary canal propelled by a series of muscle contractions called **peristalsis**.

What causes an increase in peristalsis in one part of the alimentary canal often causes the same reaction in other parts. Let's say you are taking a drug that relaxes the muscles in your colon as a side effect. That can cause constipation. But it can also cause heartburn because the muscle that keeps digestive juice in the stomach also relaxes, causing a burning splash.

Peristalsis, Fiber, and Water

The large colon is divided into four parts: the ascending, transverse, descending, and sigmoid segments. The ascending colon receives the watery chyme with undigested fiber from the small intestine. Together with the transverse colon, it reabsorbs electrolytes and water at the rate of two liters per day. How fast the chyme moves through these sections determines its water content. If the chyme moves too slow, more water is absorbed and the feces are very dry (constipation). If it moves too fast, the water does not have time to be reabsorbed and the feces are too watery (diarrhea).

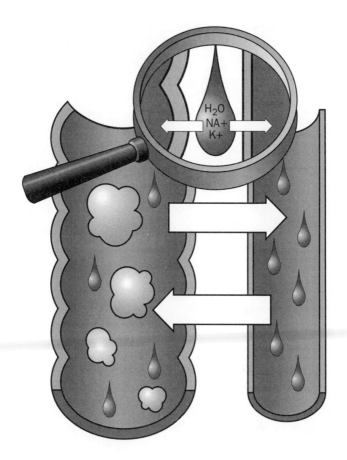

Absorption and secretion

As the peristaltic movements of the colon move the dehydrating mass along, water is trapped by the undigested fiber (primarily insoluble fibers) in the chyme, preventing the stool from becoming too dry. Other undigested fibers (primarily soluble fibers) are eaten by the many species of "friendly" bacteria that live in the colon, causing a population explosion that contributes additional bulk to the dehydrated feces.

The descending and sigmoid colons are used for storage. When fecal matter is pushed into the rectum, the distention stimulates the reflex to defecate.

Constipation

Causes of Constipation

- *Treatment Side Effects*—The toxic effects of chemotherapy, radiation, and surgery can cause problems such as sore or dry mouth and throat, difficulty in swallowing, nausea and vomiting, and lack of appetite. These side effects often greatly reduce the amount of fibrous foods you want to eat, causing constipation. In addition, the drugs used to treat side effects may further increase the chances. For example, opioid painkillers can reduce peristalsis, as

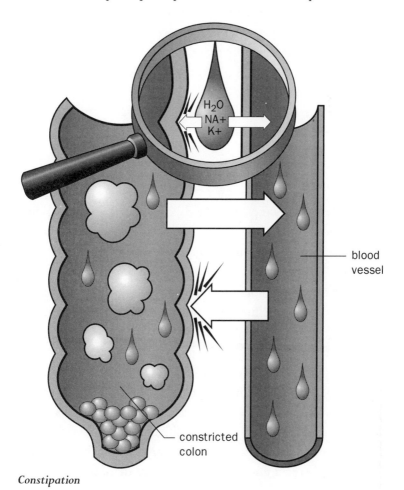

blood
vessel

constricted
colon

Constipation

can the anticholinergic drugs used to treat vomiting and diarrhea.

- *Decrease in activity*—Cancer treatment often leaves a person feeling drained and tired. Exercise becomes a low priority, and all of the muscles in the body suffer, including those responsible for colonic movement.

- *Stress*—Causes the "fight or flight" response. The body thinks it is under attack and prepares itself for hard physical exertion. Organ systems not needed for immediate use, including the digestive system, are temporarily shut down, and excess baggage is cast aside. In the case of the gastrointestinal tract, the stomach empties itself by vomiting and the colon by diarrhea. Food in the small intestine that cannot be expelled is held until normal functioning returns.

- *Loss of nerve function in the colonic muscles*—Radiation and surgery can sometimes result in a temporary or permanent loss of muscle tone due to nerve damage.

Solutions

The following dietary suggestions can help prevent or cure constipation:

- Wheat bran is the usual recommendation for increasing fiber intake, but rice bran tastes and works better. For a morning treat, sprinkle wheat bran, rice bran or polish, or ground psyllium seed on cooked or cold breakfast cereals, nonfat yogurt, or fresh fruit. Start with one teaspoon and gradually work up to a tablespoon. These foods are concentrated sources of insoluble fiber, which will increase the bulk and frequency of bowel movements by attracting water into the feces. Wheat bran holds three times its weight in water, and rice bran may hold even more. Soluble bran such as oat bran also may be effective.

- Increase the amount of water you are drinking to at least eight glasses a day. This is particularly important if you are supplementing with brans. Measure out the water in the morning so you will know how much you need to drink.

Words to Know

Diarrhea—Watery stools.
Peristalsis—Muscular contractions of the gastrointestinal tract that move food along.
Enteritis—Inflammation of the lining of the intestines.

- Increase dietary fiber. Substitute whole grains for refined grains, including brown rice for white rice and whole-grain bread for white bread. Eat a variety of grains, including oats, barley, and quinoa. Each grain has its own unique blend of fibers with unique advantages. The brans in these grains are also important sources of valuable minerals. Grainwise, brown is always better.
- Increase the amount of raw vegetables you eat. Take small bites and chew them thoroughly. If chewing is a problem, grate or blend raw veggies. If you have a juice extractor, use it to finely grate vegetables by recombining the juice and pulp after juicing.
- Eat more vegetables in the cabbage family, including bok choy, brussels sprouts, cauliflower, collards, and broccoli, and in the legume family, including beans and lentils. The gas they produce will help to increase volume and softness of bowel movements.
- Nuts and seeds are not only high in fiber, they are also rich sources of healthy fats. If you need to increase calories and fiber, eat at least two servings a day. Nuts can be whole or ground into nut butters (easy to eat if you have a sore mouth or throat). Pass on the salted or oil-roasted varieties. Nuts fresh from the shell are always best.

- Add laxative foods to your diet. Prunes and prune juice are good sources of sorbitol, a natural laxative, as are apple and pear juice.
- One cup of coffee in the morning may act as a laxative, but too much can overstimulate the muscles of the colon, leaving them sluggish. Coffee also acts as a diuretic, drawing water out of the colon, dehydrating the stool. Moderation is the key here. Limit coffee to one cup.
- Eliminate milk and cheese. These foods can cause constipation in some individuals.
- Drink hot or warm liquids before a meal to stimulate gastrointestinal tract movement.

The following home remedies may also help:
- Moving the external muscles of your body is one way to stimulate the muscles inside. Ask your doctor or nurse which kind of exercise is best for you. Even a light walk can be helpful.
- Laughing is another wonderful source of exercise. A deep belly laugh not only stimulates abdominal muscles, it also increases endorphins, the feel-good chemicals in the brain.
- Massage the abdominal muscles.

Diarrhea

Causes of Diarrhea

- *Chemotherapy* sometimes has a toxic effect on the lining of the small intestine. Some chemotherapeutic drugs can injure the villi, preventing absorption of some nutrients, and they can damage the microvilli, decreasing the amount of enzymes produced for digestion. In the large intestine some drugs increase the rate of peristalsis and the transit time through the colon, resulting in less time for water to be reabsorbed.

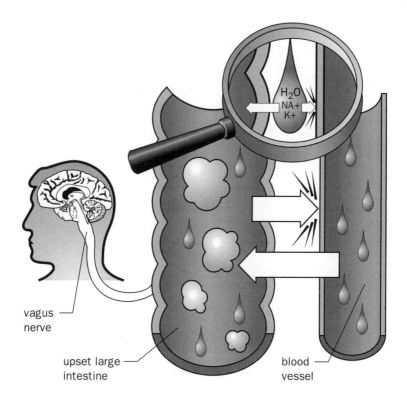

vagus
nerve

upset large
intestine

blood
vessel

Diarrhea

- *Radiation* directed to any part of the intestinal tract can cause damage to the villi of the small intestine and a decrease in repair and replacement of the injured cells. This results in loss of digestive enzymes, causing undigested food to move into the colon where it encourages diarrhea.
- *Diet*—A change in diet can cause loose stools, and some foods are notorious for this ability. A temporary intolerance to milk sugar can cause diarrhea, as can some antacids.

Solutions

Avoid the following foods, which may aggravate diarrhea:

- Hot foods stimulate muscle movement and may increase diarrhea. Try foods and beverages that are cold or at room temperature.
- Milk and other dairy products can cause diarrhea due to a temporary absence of lactase, the enzyme that digests lactose (milk sugar). Take lactase in pill form (available at your pharmacy or local health food store) before eating. Or follow the lactose-free diet described in Chapter 25.
- Avoid raw foods. Steam or pressure-cook vegetables.
- Avoid irritating foods such as coffee, alcohol, sweets, carbonated drinks, and highly spiced foods.
- Calorie-free carbonated drinks are not good sources of liquids, since they contain no energy sources or minerals to replace those in lost fluids. Sports drinks and fruit juices contain too much sugar, which can aggravate diarrhea.
- Avoid prunes and prune juice, apple juice, and pear juice. They all can have a laxative effect.
- Avoid foods that contain sorbitol, a natural laxative, including sugar-free and dietetic candies.
- Avoid foods that cause gas and are not well absorbed, such as beans and vegetables of the cabbage family (broccoli, cauliflower, kale, cabbage, and so on).

The following recommendations can help you choose foods to eat when you have diarrhea:
- Drink or eat starchy liquids such as a low-sodium split-pea or potato soup, rice or oat porridge, and mashed ripe bananas.
- The recommendation for diarrhea used to be a clear diet to rest the bowel. However, we now know that, instead of resting the bowel, this advice starves the bowel and therefore the body. Especially during treatment, the body needs nutrients to counteract the effects of the treat-

ment and keep the body fighting the cancer. Stimulation from food is necessary to keep the colon working. Disuse will cause your villi to atrophy.

- Soy protein may protect against chemotherapy-induced diarrhea. Protein powders that contain only soy protein and soymilk are convenient forms of soy protein.
- Eat a cup of nonfat yogurt. It is a natural source of friendly bacteria and a natural antibiotic. Make sure that the yogurt contains live cultures. This will be stated on the container.
- Nutmeg reduces peristalsis. Add a liberal sprinkle to a cup of yogurt or a mashed banana.
- To replenish lost potassium, eat more high-potassium foods such as bananas and potatoes.

Part III

Diet Plans: Developing Your Nutritional Therapy Regime

*C*ancer and cancer treatments can deplete the body's nutrients and cause weight loss by decreasing appetite and the body's ability to digest and absorb nutrients. At the same time, cancer speeds the metabolic rate, increasing the need for nutrients.

A balanced supplemented diet with adequate calories and protein can provide these extra nutrients. Healthy cell regeneration will reduce all cancer therapy side effects and keep the immune system functioning at its highest level.

The following diets take into consideration the common problems that many cancer patients encounter during treatment and recovery. The extra nutrients in these diets will help you to fend off weakness, repair tissue damage, boost the immune system, and generally aid in the healing process. The cancer therapy diets in this part address these issues:

- *Altered taste and smell*—Tumor growth itself, radiation, and chemotherapy treatments all have the potential to alter the ability to taste and smell. Foods may taste bitter or metallic. This change may lead to appetite loss, which in turn reduces nutrient intake, resulting in weight loss and ultimately malnutrition.

- *Anorexia*—A number of treatment side effects—loss of taste, nausea, diarrhea, and vomiting—can cause loss of appetite. Even though it may be difficult, try to eat as much as you can. Remember, if you do not use your gut, you will lose your gut. Malnutrition will decrease the amount of digestive enzymes available and decrease the absorptive area of the small intestine if food can get digested.

- *Blood sugar disorders*—Stabilizing blood sugar is critical in controlling cancer. High blood sugar levels (hyperglycemia) and low blood sugar levels (hypoglycemia) stress the immune system, weakening your ability to heal. Cancer cells need glucose for fuel and will alter the body's metabolism to keep blood sugar levels high. Starve your tumor by eliminating refined dietary sugars and increasing fiber.
- *Food allergens*—Avoid food allergens, as food allergies may be exacerbated by cancer treatments. Eat a variety of foods to avoid developing a sensitivity to any particular food.
- *Malabsorption*—Food may not be absorbed properly through the intestines into the bloodstream. For example, each segment of the intestines absorbs different nutrients. Surgery to remove part of the intestine dramatically affects the body's ability to absorb the corresponding nutrients. Pancreatic cancer can cause a decrease in insulin production, affecting carbohydrate metabolism. Radiation or surgery of the intestines or other areas of the abdomen can cause diarrhea, cramps, or decreased absorption.
- *Maldigestion*—The body's ability to produce digestive enzymes and break down foods for absorption may be reduced by the stress of illness. Signals that normally stimulate your appetite may not be functioning. This can cause the stomach not to release digestive juices.
- *Mechanical difficulties*—Difficulty in chewing and swallowing may be the result of tumors in the head or neck area or an aftereffect of surgery.
- *Weight loss cycle*—Decreased appetite and the resulting weight loss can lead to fatigue and depression. This, in turn, leads to less activity and even more weight loss. Soon the body's resistance to disease and ability to heal decline as well. Lower resistance may affect the amount

of chemotherapy or radiation treatment that can be delivered, hindering your healing process.

It is best to start these diets before treatment begins. They are designed to increase your nutrient stores and prepare the body for the friendly fire of cancer treatment.

See page 265 for a Nutrition Treatment Plan checklist. Use this checklist as a starting point for discussion about your treatment plan with your physician and other practitioners.

20

The Basic Diet

The diet described in this chapter is for those just diagnosed who have no symptoms and are otherwise healthy.

The healthiest diet for anyone is a whole-foods diet based on a menu of whole grains, legumes, fruits, vegetables, and fish that are as unprocessed and as unrefined as possible. Whole foods are nutrient dense, full of fiber, and have minimal chemicals and additives. Buying organic produce will reduce your exposure to chemicals even further. Eating a variety of whole foods will ensure you are getting a wide variety of nutrients to build healthy new cells and to provide brain food and a daily ration of energy calories.

Any illness and its treatments will tax nutrient supplies, creating a need to supplement the diet with the micronutrients—vitamins and minerals. Dietary intake of fat, carbohydrate, and protein must meet the body's requirements for healing and functioning. If you are not able to take in these nutrients through the diet, a supplemental program may be necessary. It is vital to avoid malnutrition through a proper diet.

Ideally whole foods should be made at home, where relaxation and enjoyment of the eating experience is the fullest. If ordering healthful food from restaurants or going out to eat are pleasurable experiences, then these also are options. If cooking is impossible because you are exhausted or weak, yet financial restrictions eliminate the restaurant fare, there are inexpensive food delivery programs such as "Meals on Wheels" to get food to cancer patients. For information on such programs, consult the resources appendix in the back of this book.

The Diet Plan

This is a whole-foods diet: high in vegetable protein and fiber and low in total fat and saturated fat. It emphasizes nutritionally dense foods such as beans, peas, lentils, vegetables, fruits, nuts, seeds, and food supplements to increase nutrient stores, strengthen the immune system, and weaken the tumor before cancer treatment begins.

Macronutrient Guidelines

- 30 percent fat (from fish, poultry, flaxseed, fish oil, and olive oil)
- 55 percent complex carbohydrate (from whole grains, legumes, and vegetables)
- 15 to 20 percent protein (from beans, peas, and lentils)
- Eight to ten 8-ounce glasses of water each day (preferably filtered)

To know if you are consuming enough protein and calories, perform the following calculations:

Desirable weight: _____ pounds
    (See chart and fill in your weight.)
Minimum daily protein requirement =
    Desirable weight $\times$ 0.5 = _____ grams
Daily calorie requirement (for men) =
    Desirable weight $\times$ 18 = _____ calories
Daily calorie requirement (for women) =
    Desirable weight $\times$ 16 = _____ calories

Meal Planning

- Eat five to six small meals rather than two to three large ones.
- If you cannot manage to eat all of the recommended vegetable servings, try juicing some of them.
- Foods that taste sweet should be eaten only on a full stomach.

U.S. Department of Agriculture, U.S. Department of Health and Human Services Acceptable Weights for Adults

Weight in Pounds†‡

HEIGHT*	19 TO 34 YEARS	35 YEARS AND OVER
5'0"	97–128	108–138
5'1"	101–132	111–143
5'2"	104–137	115–148
5'3"	107–141	119–152
5'4"	111–146	122–157
5'5"	114–150	126–162
5'6"	118–155	130–167
5'7"	121–160	134–172
5'8"	125–164	138–178
5'9"	129–169	142–183
5'10"	132–174	146–188
5'11"	136–179	151–194
6'0"	140–184	155–199
6'1"	144–189	159–205
6'2"	148–195	164–210
6'3"	152–200	168–216
6'4"	156–205	173–222
6'5"	160–211	177–228
6'6"	164–216	182–234

*Without shoes.

†Without clothes.

‡The higher weights in the ranges generally apply to men, who tend to have more muscle and bone; the lower weights more often apply to women, who have less muscle and bone.

From Human Nutrition Information Service. U.S. Department of Agriculture. Report of the Dietary Guidelines Advisory Committee on the dietary guidelines for Americans—1990. Hyattsville, MD: U.S. Government Printing Office, June, 1990:8.

- Cook meals that are appealing to the eye as well as the palate.
- Drink eight to ten glasses of water (preferably filtered) a day.
- Whenever you are hungry, snack on high-protein foods. A handful of nuts is a good choice.
- Don't drink fluids or soups before or with meals. They will fill you up and leave no room for foods that are nutrient dense.
- Make mealtimes a pleasant experience by relaxing before a meal, eating with friends or family, and creating a pleasant atmosphere at the table.
- If you lose weight, increase serving sizes. If you gain weight, decrease serving sizes.

A 5 percent loss from your normal weight is considered significant. Losing 10 percent of your normal weight should be considered a red flag. A 15 percent weight loss may lead to loss of appetite, fatigue, depression, and reduced ability to heal.

If you aren't getting enough calories, proteins, and nutrients from this whole-foods diet and do not gain and maintain the proper weight, a nutritional supplement may be necessary. We prefer homemade protein shakes and a multivitamin to the canned liquid supplements.

Basic Supplement Regime

Along with the foods recommended, take the following supplements each day:

- *Vitamin E*—Take 1,600 IU as mixed tocopherols. Get part from the multivitamin and the remainder from the antioxidant supplement.
- *Vitamin K*—Take this vitamin as part of a multivitamin supplement. Large doses of vitamin E require extra vitamin K.
- *Mixed carotenes*—Take 100,000 IU as mixed carotenes. Get

part from the multivitamin and the remainder from the antioxidant supplement.

- *Multivitamin/mineral formula*—Take the "optimal" recommended dosage stated on the bottle.
- *Antioxidant formula*—This should contain vitamin C, vitamin E, beta-carotene and mixed carotenes, and selenium. Some comprehensive formulas also contain green tea extract and silymarin.
- *Fish oil (EPA)*—Take 1,000 to 1,600 milligrams EPA as fish oil. The amount per capsule and gram of fish oil differs depending on the source. Check the bottle for EPA levels.

Warning: When supplementing any fat-soluble vitamin or oil, you must also take a vitamin E supplement to protect against oxidation.

Foods to Eat Every Day

Include the minimum number of servings every day. Some days your average serving size will be smaller, and other days it will be larger. Remember, the *number* of servings is more important than the *size* of the servings.

Cruciferous Vegetables
at least 2 servings a day (One serving may be juiced.)

broccoli	kale
brussels sprouts	collard and mustard
cabbage	greens
bok choy	cauliflower

Serving Suggestions: Add cruciferous vegetables to casseroles or salads. Sauté with tofu and seeds. Mix ¼ cup olive oil with ¼ cup balsamic vinegar and 2 tablespoons sesame seeds; sprinkle over the top of raw chopped cabbage and cauliflower. Steam brussels sprouts and top with a shaving of butter. Dip cauliflower heads into ranch dressing for a light snack.

What Is One Serving?

These are the average serving sizes. If you cannot eat this amount of food when you are in therapy, decrease the size but not the number of servings. Variety of food is more important than quantity of food.

In the beginning, always measure your food. You may think you are using one cup, but it may be more or less.

Bread, Cereal, Rice, and Pasta

1 slice bread
1 ounce ready-to-eat cereal (Check labels: 1 ounce equals ¼ cup to 2 cups, depending on the cereal.)
½ cup cooked cereal, rice, or pasta
½ bagel or English muffin
3 or 4 plain crackers (small)

Vegetables

1 cup raw leafy vegetables
½ cup other vegetables, cooked or chopped raw
½ cup fresh vegetable juice

Fruit

1 medium apple, banana, orange, nectarine, or peach
½ cup chopped, cooked, or dried fruit
¾ cup fruit juice

Milk, Yogurt, and Cheese

1 cup milk or yogurt
1½ ounces natural cheese (a thin slice or 1-inch cube)

Poultry, Fish, Beans, Eggs, and Nuts

2–3 ounces cooked poultry or fish (about the size of a deck of cards)
1 cup cooked beans
1 egg
2 tablespoons nut butter
A handful of seeds or shelled nuts

Fats and Oils

2 teaspoons vegetable or nut oil
2 teaspoons butter
2 teaspoons mayonnaise
1 tablespoon oil- or mayonnaise-based salad dressing

Antioxidant Vegetables
at least 1 – 2 servings a day (One serving may be juiced.)

yams	tomatoes
sweet potatoes	bell peppers
carrots	asparagus
spinach	

Serving Suggestions: Steam, bake, pressure-cook, or sauté with 1 tablespoon olive oil. Stuff baked veggies with grains or beans.

Green Leafy Vegetables
1 – 2 servings a day

Swiss chard	escarole
dark green lettuces	chicory
(green and red	dandelion greens
loose-leaf, romaine,	sprouts
butter)	sorrel

Green vegetables are carotene-rich foods containing beta-carotene, other carotenoids, and vitamin C, which act as free radical scavengers, immune stimulators, and may even be toxic to tumors. Consistent epidemiological findings show a strong association between high beta-carotene intake and reduced incidence of squamous cell carcinomas, even in smokers. They also contain cancer-fighting phytochemicals such as calcium, indoles, phthalides, ellagic acid, and flavonoids. Green leafy vegetables contain soluble and insoluble fiber, which increases stool bulk and dilutes possible harmful substances in the intestinal tract.

Serving Suggestions: Steam vegetables or sauté with 1 tablespoon extra-virgin olive oil and 1 teaspoon sesame seeds. Serve with a splash of tamari or soy sauce. Green leafy vegetables cook quickly; steam or sauté for just 1–2 minutes. Serve with tofu or bean dishes.

Other Vegetables

1 serving a day (optional)

potatoes

rutabaga

turnips

beets

winter and summer
    squash

cucumbers

pumpkin

corn

green beans

wax beans

snow peas

sea vegetables (kelp,

kombu, wakame,

agar-agar, dulse,

carrageenan

(Irish moss), nori,

sea lettuce, or

supplement)

mushrooms (shiitake,

maitake, Reishi, or

mushroom extract)

radishes

okra

kohlrabi

water chestnuts

Sea vegetables contain thyroid-stimulating substances and are loaded with the minerals calcium, potassium, iron, phosphorus, and iodine. They are high in fiber, low in fat, and contain vitamins A and B complex, as well as small quantities of vitamin C.

Serving Suggestions: Steam, stir-fry, sauté, or layer in a casserole. Add raw vegetables to vegetable sandwiches. Juice them or cook them in soup. Sea vegetables can be crushed or chopped and added to soups, stews, stir-fry, or salads.

Fruit

at least 2 servings a day with meals, including 1 citrus (One serving may be juiced.)

citrus fruits (oranges,
lemons, grapefruit,
tangerines)
other fresh fruits
(bananas, plums,
peaches, apricots,
cherries, apples,
berries, cantaloupe,
mango, papaya, pears,
strawberries,
watermelon)
dried fruit (figs, dates,
raisins, prunes)
stewed fruit (applesauce)

Dried fruits offer concentrated amounts of vitamins, minerals, and fiber while satisfying the sweet tooth. Drink water with these foods to help with digestion. Avoid those treated with sulfur or other preservatives.

Serving Suggestions: Eat fruit only with meals. Remove skin, if fruit is not organic, to remove any pesticide residue. Fruits can be served raw, steamed, or baked. Baked pears with a sprinkle of cinnamon and a drizzle of honey are easy to digest, and the aroma of baking fruit is an appetite stimulant.

Legumes

2 – 3 servings a day (This can include one of the soyfood servings.)

beans (soybeans, adzuki
beans, lima beans,
black beans, black-
eyed peas, brown
beans, pinto beans,
red beans, fava beans,
kidney beans, navy
beans, white beans,
chickpeas)
lentils
split peas
green peas

Beans, peas, and lentils contain protease inhibitors, which inhibit tumor growth. They contain complex carbohydrate for pure energy food and are the perfect high-fiber, low-fat protein food. The fiber binds with toxins in the colon and cleans them out before they can be reabsorbed. The slowly metabolized carbohydrates release glucose gradually into the bloodstream, which makes them the ideal food for stabilizing blood sugar. Soybeans, for example, contain isoflavones and phytoestrogens, powerful anticancer phytochemicals.

Serving Suggestions: Dried legumes can take a long time to cook and usually require soaking overnight and cooking for 1 hour or more, depending on the type of bean. A pressure cooker allows you to skip the overnight soak and shortens the cooking time to about 30 minutes. Legumes can be added to soups, stews, and casseroles or served cold in salads or as dips. Digestive enzymes such as Beano can be used to aid in digestion and reduce the gas-forming effects of all beans.

Nuts and Seeds
at least 1 serving a day

fresh nuts (almonds, Brazil nuts, cashews, filberts, pecans, pine nuts, pistachios, and walnuts)
fresh unseasoned seeds (pumpkin seeds, sesame seeds, sunflower seeds, flaxseed)
nut and seed butters (tahini or sesame seed butter, walnut butter, almond butter, hazelnut butter, cashew butter, sunflower butter)
nut milks

Nuts and seeds are excellent sources of protein and fiber. They are also high in heart-healthy fats and contain no cholesterol. For those wishing to gain weight, nuts and seeds and their butters are a high-calorie protein source. Enjoy them raw or roasted and unsalted.

Serving Suggestions: Nuts can be eaten whole as snacks, added to salads, or cooked with vegetables. Add nut butters to sauces and soups, or use as spreads in sandwiches or on crackers.

Soy Products
at least 1 serving a day

soymilk (regular,
  low-fat, nonfat,
  fortified, vanilla,
  chocolate, carob)
tofu
tempeh

soy nuts
soy flour
soy grits
soy cheese
soybeans
miso

One cup of soybeans contains twenty-eight grams of protein (half the RDA), fiber, zinc, B vitamins, half a day's supply of iron, and loads of highly absorbable calcium. Soy appears to have many benefits in the treatment of cancer. Soy products inhibit breast cancer by decreasing estrogen levels. Soy blocks the cancer-promoting action of natural estrogens. One serving a day of soy may decrease the risk of developing a number of cancers by nearly 40 percent. Soy also has a cholesterol-lowering effect. Soybeans contain phytoesterols, which help protect against heart disease and are effective against skin cancer. Soy contains saponins, which are antioxidants and play a role in cancer prevention. High levels of estrogen are linked to increased risk of breast cancer and other hormone-related cancers. Isoflavones are antiestrogens and act as protectors against elevated estrogen cancers.

Genistein, an isoflavone found in soy products, is protective against leukemia and cancer of the colon, breast, lung, prostate, and skin. Oncogenes produce enzymes that can cause our cells to mutate dangerously and become cancer cells. One of those dangerous enzymes produced by the oncogenes is tyrosine protein kinase, a cell growth stimulator. Genistein is a potent inhibitor of tyrosine protein kinases, and it also appears to be an effective anticarcinogen against other enzymes involved in the cancer process. Soy also contains protease inhibitors, which appear to inhibit or prevent cancer growth.

Serving Suggestions: Soymilk is an easy, delicious way to put soyfoods into your diet. Use soymilk on cereals, in hot drinks, and in cooking. Make soymilk smoothies or scrambled tofu instead of eggs. (Sauté ½ chopped onion in 1 tablespoon olive oil. Add 16 ounces crumbled firm tofu and sauté until heated through. Sprinkle top with turmeric powder and soy sauce and serve.) Make soy cheese sandwiches, crumble tofu to replace tuna or egg in a tuna or egg salad sandwich, snack on soy nuts, and add cubes of miso to soups. For a healthful dip, combine 16 ounces tofu and 1 avocado in the blender. Use tofu in place of hamburger in tacos; add the taco seasoning directly to sautéed tofu. Blend silken tofu into creamed soups, cream sauces, and puddings or pie fillings instead of evaporated milk. Marinate strips of tofu with tamari, honey, sesame seeds, and fresh ginger to eat cold as snacks. Slice tempeh and brush top with barbecue sauce for a grilled meal. Miso can be used as a flavoring agent or to make quick soups.

Grains

at least 6–11 servings a day

whole grains (amaranth, barley, buckwheat, corn, kamut, millet, oats, quinoa, brown rice, rye, spelt, triticale, wheat, wild rice)
whole-grain products (pasta, breads, crackers, flours, unsalted air-popped popcorn)
cereals (hot and cold with no added sugar)
brans (oat, rice, wheat)
germs (wheat, rice polish)

Each whole grain has its own unique combination of vitamins, minerals, fibers, and phytochemicals. Whole grains and their brans and germs are excellent sources of the B vitamins, vitamin E, and protein, as well as the minerals calcium, iron, magnesium, phosphorus, potassium, selenium, and zinc. Both rice and wheat bran are excellent sources of the insoluble fiber necessary for colon health. Remember to always eat a vitamin C source with whole grains to increase mineral absorption.

Serving Suggestions: Whole-grain pastas, and hot cereals such as nine-grain or steel cut oats are easy ways to put more grain variety into your diet. Serve these cereals with rice, soy, or almond milk. For hot savory meals, cook grain dishes like brown rice, teff, amaranth, millet, quinoa, spelt, or wild rice. Cold grain salads such as tabbouleh, kamut salad, or bulgur can be soothing to the throat. Cooking the grains in a vegetable or nonfat chicken broth adds depth of flavor without irritating seasonings that may be too strong after chemotherapy.

Cook whole grains well and serve with vegetables or beans. Add them to soups or casseroles, and use flours to make chipatis, breads, cakes, or pie crusts. Whole-grain products such as crackers, pastas, and breads are now available. Grain products such as bulgur (cracked wheat), semolina (wheat pasta pellets), and cornmeal can be cooked as you would whole grains. These products contain delicate oils, so they must be refrigerated in airtight containers to retain their nutrient value and to keep them from becoming rancid.

Dairy products
at least 1 serving a day

yogurt (low-fat, nonfat,
    plain, flavored)
milk (nonfat and
    skim unflavored,
    buttermilk,

acidophilus, nonfat
    powdered or instant)
cottage cheese (nonfat,
    low-fat)

Yogurt is milk treated with healthy strains of bacteria such as *Lactobacillus bulgaricus*, *Lactobacillus acidophilus*, and *Streptococcus thermophilus*. It provides protein, calcium, and other vitamins and minerals. The bacteria in yogurt promote the regrowth of the healthy microflora in the gut after they have been killed by antibiotics, chemotherapeutic agents, or radiation. A healthy balance of intestinal bacteria is important for proper digestion of fiber and absorption of vitamins. Yogurt that contains live cultures will have this fact marked on the label; look for it.

Serving Suggestions: Top bean and rice dishes with a dollop of yogurt. Use yogurt as a base for shakes and smoothies or in place of sour cream or mayonnaise in dips and dressings.

Seasonings
use liberally

garlic, onions, leeks, and scallions (raw and cooked)

gingerroot (juiced, raw, brewed)

hot peppers (dried, raw, cooked)

rosemary

curry

cumin

basil

caraway seeds

cloves

tarragon

turmeric

Fats and Oils
up to 1 serving a day

canola oil

olive oil

nut oils (walnut, macadamia, almond)

salad dressings (canola oil mayonnaise, dressings made with olive or canola oil)

Beverages

as desired

tea (green, black)
herbal teas (any
  unsweetened)
filtered water
ginger tea

coffee substitutes
  (Cafix, Postum,
  Roma, chicory, or
  roasted barley drinks)
rice milk

Foods to Eat Weekly (Optional)

Butter

2 – 3 servings a week

butter (salted, unsalted,
  whipped)

Dairy Products

1 – 2 servings a week

cheese, low-fat cream
  cheese
sour cream

evaporated or
  condensed milk

Serving Suggestions: Add cheese to sauces, serve over vegetables, with crackers, in casseroles, on potatoes, layered in lasagna and as between-meal snacks. Eat cheese only if you are not having a problem with lactose intolerance or mucus formation.

Eggs

up to 6 a week

cooked eggs

Serving Suggestions: Add hard-boiled eggs to salads and sandwiches. Use eggs in sauces, omelets, breads, and soups. Never eat raw or undercooked eggs.

Poultry and Fish

3 – 5 servings a week

skinless fresh poultry
(turkey, chicken,
game hens)
cooked fish (especially

fatty fish such as
salmon, mackerel,
herring)

Serving Suggestions: Use poultry as a condiment. Add to sandwiches, soups, and salads or stir-fry.

Peanuts

1 serving a week

roasted, fresh, unsalted
peanuts

peanut butter

Peanut butter is not recommended as an everyday food because high levels of aflatoxins normally are present. Overconsumption of aflatoxins has been known to be carcinogenic. However, many other nut butters do not have high levels of aflatoxins.

Serving Suggestions: Eat peanut butter on toast, in cookies, on celery, on crackers, or on a spoon.

Sweets

2 – 3 times a week

unrefined sweeteners
(grain syrups, maple
syrup, honey, and
Sucanat)
diluted fruit juices
(fresh, frozen,
bottled)
hard candies

chocolate
sweetened cocoa
frozen desserts (ice
milk, frozen yogurt,
sorbet, sherbet, juice
pops)
fruit spreads and
preserves

Never eat sweets on an empty stomach. Always eat them as part of a meal.

Foods to Avoid

Coffee

caffeine-free coffee

regular coffee

instant coffee

flavored coffee

drip coffee

lattes and other
espresso drinks

iced coffee

Sweetened Drinks

all bottled or
canned soft drinks
(regular, diet, and
caffeine-free)

bottled and canned
iced teas

juice-flavored drinks

(such as Sunny
Delight)

powdered instant drinks
(including sweetened
or unsweetened
Kool-Aid, lemonade)

canned juices

Candy

candy bars

granola bars

fruit roll-ups

chocolate-covered fruit

Smoked, Cured, or Pickled Foods

bacon

hot dogs

smoked luncheon meats

pepperoni and other
smoked sausages

ham

Spam

canned meat spreads

pickled eggs

pickles

pickled herring

Meat

beef

buffalo

pork

ham

bacon

processed meats

liver

heart

tripe

pig's feet

Raw Animal Foods
raw or undercooked
   eggs
sushi (raw fish)

any other raw animal
   food

Refined or Processed Foods
white sugar
white-flour products
   (pancake mixes, cake
   mixes, pudding
   mixes)
refined cereals
white bread

cakes
pies
gelatins
prepared puddings
yogurts with candy
   stir-ins

Salty Foods
potato chips
corn chips
pretzels
theater-style popcorn

canned regular soups
high-sodium seasonings
any other salty food

Dairy Products
high-fat milk products
   (whole milk, cream,
   half-and-half,
   chocolate milk, milk
   shakes)

whole yogurt
yogurt with stir-in
   candies or sweetened
   cereals
yogurt with aspartame

Fatty Foods
deep-fried foods (french
   fries, fried fish,
   tempura, doughnuts)

fast food (hamburgers,
   hot dogs, fried pies)
grilled meat
poultry skin

Alcohol

whiskey	gin
rum	wine
bourbon	beer
tequila	liqueurs

Spreads

margarine or oleo	oil spreads
butter substitutes	low-fat spreads

Artificial Sweeteners

aspartame	any food or drink
NutraSweet	containing these
Equal	products
saccharin	

Fat Substitutes

Olestra	any food or drink
Simpless	containing these
	products

Vegetable Oils and Saturated Fats

corn oil	suet
soybean oil	vegetable shortening
lard	

21

Underweight Diet Plan

*I*f you are underweight when diagnosed with cancer, this is the diet plan for you to follow.

People can be thin for many reasons. Sometimes they are just naturally thin and have a high metabolism. Other times it is the result of dieting to keep weight at a socially accept-able level, a sign of malabsorption, or an indication of mal-nutrition. If you have trouble gaining or maintaining weight, see your doctor. You may have a thyroid problem or a disease that causes malabsorption, such as celiac disease.

While a thin, underweight body is much admired in the fashion magazines, it is often not strong enough to withstand the rigors of cancer and cancer treatment. Low weight means low levels of lean muscle tissue, low stores of fat for days when you cannot eat, and low stores of vitamins and minerals such as vitamin A, iron, and calcium.

If you are on a diet and eating less than 1,200 calories a day, stop. It is impossible to get all of the nutrients you need to prepare your body for treatment on this small amount of food. Remember, you are essentially preparing for war, and a store-house of nutrients will be necessary to feed your immune soldiers.

On the other hand, don't just stuff yourself with anything that will fit in your mouth. Fried pies and Twinkies will cause a weight gain, but not the type you need. Junk food will put fat on you, but it will do nothing for building nutrient stores and building lean muscle tissue.

This diet is designed to build you up without building you out. It should result in a modest weight gain that allows you to put on some fat stores.

The Diet Plan

This is a whole-foods diet designed to encourage your body to gain weight. It is high in vegetable protein and fiber and low in saturated fat. This plan emphasizes nutritionally dense high-fat foods such as nuts, seeds, and food supplements to increase fat and protein stores, strengthen the immune system, and weaken the tumor before cancer treatment begins.

Macronutrient Guidelines

- 25 to 30 percent calories from fat (from fish, poultry, flaxseed, fish oil, and olive oil)
- 55 percent calories from complex carbohydrate (from whole grains, legumes, fruits, and vegetables)
- 15 to 20 percent calories from protein (from legumes, nuts and seeds, soyfoods, and lentils)
- Eight to ten 8-ounce glasses of water each day (preferably filtered)

To know if you are consuming enough protein and calories, perform the following calculations:

Desirable weight: _____ pounds
 (See chart in chapter 20 and fill in your weight.)
Minimum daily protein requirement =
 Desirable weight × 0.5 = _____ grams
Daily calorie requirement (for men) =
 Desirable weight × 18 = _____ calories
Daily calorie requirement (for women) =
 Desirable weight × 16 = _____ calories

Meal Planning

- Eat five to six small meals rather than two to three large ones.
- If you cannot manage to eat all of the recommended vegetable servings, try juicing some of them.

- Foods that taste sweet should be eaten only on a full stomach.
- Cook meals that are appealing to the eye as well as the palate.
- Drink eight to ten glasses of water (preferably filtered) a day.
- Read Chapter 17 regarding appetite loss and follow the guidelines there.
- Whenever you are hungry, snack on high-protein foods. A handful of nuts is a good choice.
- Half an hour before meals, drink half a glass of water with a teaspoon of lemon juice to stimulate digestive juices.
- Exercise about half an hour before meals to stimulate the appetite.
- Don't drink fluids or soups before or with meals. They will fill you up and leave no room for foods that are nutrient dense.
- Make mealtimes a pleasant experience by relaxing before the meal, eating with friends or family, and creating a pleasant atmosphere at the table.
- If you do not gain weight, increase serving sizes.

A 5 percent weight loss from your normal weight is considered significant. Losing 10 percent of your normal weight should be considered a red flag. A 15 percent weight loss may lead to loss of appetite, fatigue, depression, and reduced ability to heal.

If you do not obtain enough calories, proteins, and nutrients from this whole-foods diet and do not gain and maintain the proper weight, a nutritional supplement may be necessary. We prefer homemade protein shakes and a multivitamin to the canned liquid supplements.

Supplement Regime

Along with the foods recommended, take the following supplements each day:

- *Vitamin E*—Take 1,600 IU as mixed tocopherols. Get part from the multivitamin and the remainder from the antioxidant supplement.
- *Vitamin K*—Take this vitamin as part of a multivitamin supplement. Large doses of vitamin E require extra vitamin K.
- *Mixed carotenes*—Take 100,000 IU as mixed carotenes. Get part from the multivitamin and the remainder from the antioxidant supplement.
- *Multivitamin/mineral formula*—Take the "optimal" recommended dosage stated on the bottle.
- *Antioxidant formula*—This should contain vitamin C, vitamin E, beta-carotene and mixed carotenes, and selenium. Some comprehensive formulas also contain green tea extract and silymarin.
- *Fish oil (epa)*—Take 1,000–1,600 milligrams EPA as fish oil. The amount of EPA per capsule and gram of fish oil differs depending on the source. Check the bottle for EPA levels.

Warning: When supplementing any fat-soluble vitamin or oil, you must also take a vitamin E supplement to protect against oxidation.

Foods to Eat Every Day

Include the minimum number of servings every day. Some days your average serving size will be smaller, and other days it will be larger. Remember, the *number* of servings is more important than the *size* of the servings.

Cruciferous Vegetables
at least 2 servings a day (One serving may be juiced.)

broccoli	kale
brussels sprouts	collard and mustard
cabbage	greens
bok choy	cauliflower

Antioxidant Vegetables
at least 1 – 2 servings a day (One serving may be juiced.)

yams	tomatoes
sweet potatoes	bell peppers
carrots	asparagus
spinach	

Green Leafy Vegetables
1 – 2 servings a day

Swiss chard	escarole
dark green lettuces	chicory
(green and red	dandelion greens
loose-leaf, romaine,	sprouts
butter)	sorrel

What Is One Serving?

These are the average serving sizes. If you cannot eat this amount of food when you are in therapy, decrease the size but not the number of servings. Variety of food is more important than quantity of food.

In the beginning, always measure your food. You may think you are using one cup, but it may be more or less.

Bread, Cereal, Rice, and Pasta

1 slice bread
1 ounce ready-to-eat cereal (Check labels: 1 ounce equals
¼ cup to 2 cups, depending on the cereal.)
½ cup cooked cereal, rice, or pasta
½ bagel or English muffin
3 or 4 plain crackers (small)

Vegetables

1 cup raw leafy vegetables
½ cup other vegetables, cooked or chopped raw
½ cup fresh vegetable juice

Fruit

1 medium apple, banana, orange, nectarine, or peach
½ cup chopped, cooked, or dried fruit
¾ cup fruit juice

Milk, Yogurt, and Cheese

1 cup milk or yogurt
1½ ounces natural cheese (a thin slice or 1-inch cube)

Poultry, Fish, Beans, Eggs, and Nuts

2–3 ounces cooked poultry or fish (about the size of a deck of cards)
1 cup cooked beans
1 egg
2 tablespoons nut butter
A handful of seeds or shelled nuts

Fats and Oils

2 teaspoons vegetable or nut oil
2 teaspoons butter
2 teaspoons mayonnaise
1 tablespoon oil- or mayonnaise-based salad dressing

Other Vegetables
1 serving a day

potatoes
rutabaga
turnips
beets
winter and summer
  squash
cucumbers
pumpkin
corn
green beans
wax beans
sea vegetables (kelp,

kombu, wakame,
agar-agar, dulse,
carrageenan, nori,
and sea lettuce, or
  supplement)
mushrooms (shiitake,
  maitake, reishi, or
  mushroom extract)
radishes
okra
kohlrabi
water chestnuts

Fruit
2 servings a day with meals, including at least 1 citrus (One serving may be juiced.)

citrus fruits (oranges,
  lemons, grapefruit,
  tangerines)
fresh fruits (bananas,
  plums, peaches,
  apricots, cherries,
  apples, berries,

cantaloupe, apricots,
  mango, papaya, pears,
  strawberries,
  watermelon)
dried fruit (figs, dates,
  raisins, prunes)
stewed fruit (applesauce)

Legumes

2 – 3 servings a day (This can include 1 of the soy food servings.)

beans (soybeans, adzuki
  beans, lima beans,
  black beans, black-
  eyed peas, brown
  beans, pinto beans,
  red beans, fava beans,

kidney beans, navy
  beans, white beans,
  and chickpeas)
lentils and split peas
green peas

Nuts and Seeds

at least 2 servings a day

fresh nuts (almonds,
  Brazil nuts, cashews,
  filberts, pecans, pine
  nuts, pistachios, and
  walnuts)
fresh unseasoned seeds
  (pumpkin seeds,
  sesame seeds,
  sunflower seeds,

flaxseed)
nut and seed butters
  (tahini or sesame seed
  butter, walnut butter,
  almond butter,
  hazelnut butter,
  cashew butter, and
  sunflower butter)
nut milks

Soy Products

at least 1 – 2 servings a day

soymilk (regular,
  low-fat, nonfat,
  fortified, vanilla,
  chocolate, and carob)
tofu
tempeh

soy nuts
soy flour
soy grits
soy cheese
soybeans
miso

Grains

at least 6-11 servings a day

whole grains (amaranth, barley, buckwheat, corn, kamut, millet, oats, quinoa, brown rice, rye, spelt, triticale, wheat, wild rice)
whole grain products (pasta, breads, crackers, flours, unsalted air-popped popcorn)
cereals (hot and cold with no added sugar)
brans (oat, rice, wheat)
germs (wheat, rice polish)

Dairy Products

at least 1 serving a day

yogurt (low-fat, nonfat, plain, flavored)
milk (nonfat and skim unflavored, buttermilk, acidophilus, nonfat powdered or instant)
cottage cheese (nonfat)

Seasonings

use liberally

garlic, onions, leeks, and scallions (raw and cooked)
gingerroot (juiced, raw brewed)
hot peppers (dried, raw, cooked)
rosemary
curry
cumin
basil
caraway seeds
cloves
tarragon
turmeric

Fats and Oils

2 – 3 servings a day

canola oil

olive oil

nut oils (walnut, macadamia, almond)

salad dressings (canola oil mayonnaise, dressing made with olive or canola oil)

Beverages

as desired

tea (green, black)

herbal teas (any unsweetened)

filtered water

ginger tea

coffee substitutes (Cafix, Postum, Roma, chicory, or roasted barley drinks)

rice milk

Food to Eat Weekly (Optional)

Butter

2 – 3 servings a week

butter (salted, unsalted, whipped)

Dairy Products

2 – 3 times a week

cheese

low-fat cream cheese

sour cream

evaporated or condensed milk

Eggs

4 – 6 eggs a week

cooked eggs

Poultry and Fish
3 – 5 servings a week

skinless fresh poultry
(turkey, chicken,
game hens)

cooked fish (especially
fatty fish such as
salmon, mackerel,
herring)

Peanuts
1 serving a week

roasted, fresh, unsalted
peanuts

peanut butter

Sweets
1 – 2 times a week

unrefined sweeteners
(grain syrups, maple
syrup, honey, and
Sucanat)
diluted fruit juices
(fresh, frozen,
bottled)
hard candies

chocolate
sweetened cocoa
frozen desserts (ice
milk, frozen yogurt,
sorbet, sherbet, juice
pops)
fruit spreads and
preserves

Note: Never eat sweets on an empty stomach. Always eat them as part of a meal.

Wine (at physician's discretion)
1 4-ounce glass before meals once or twice a week

any dry red or
white wine

Avoid sparkling wines. The bubbles kill the appetite.

Foods to Avoid

Coffee

caffeine-free coffee
regular coffee
instant coffee
flavored coffee
drip coffee
lattes and other espresso
    drinks
iced coffee

Sweetened Drinks

all bottled or canned
    soft drinks (regular,
    diet, and caffeine-
    free)
bottled and canned iced
    teas
fruit-flavored drinks
(such as Sunny
    Delight)
powdered instant drinks
    (including sweetened
    or unsweetened Kool-
    Aid, lemonade)
canned juices

Sweets

candy bars (chocolate
    bars, including Mars,
    Snickers, M&Ms)
piece candy (Gummy
    Bears, Sweet Tarts,
    bubble gum, jelly
    beans, and the like)
granola bars (processed
    in packages)
jellies and jams
"pop-up" toaster tarts
and pastries
snack cakes (such as
    Twinkies, HoHos,
    cupcakes, handheld
    pies)
caramel corn
high-fat and sugar
    cookies
fruit roll-ups
chocolate-covered fruit
    and nuts

Salted Foods

potato chips
corn chips
pretzels
theater-style popcorn
canned regular soups
high-sodium seasonings

Smoked, Cured, or Pickled Foods

bacon	Spam
hot dogs	canned meat spreads
smoked luncheon meats	pickled eggs
pepperoni and other	pickles
smoked sausages	pickled herring
ham	

Meat

beef	processed meats
buffalo	liver
pork	heart
ham	tripe
bacon	pig's feet

Raw Animal Foods

raw or undercooked	any other raw
eggs	animal food
sushi (raw fish)	

Refined or Processed Foods

white sugar	cakes
white-flour products	pies
(pancake mixes,	gelatins
cake mixes,	prepared puddings
pudding mixes)	yogurts with candy
refined cereals	stir-ins
white bread	

Alcohol

whiskey	gin
rum	beer
bourbon	liqueurs
tequila	

Dairy Products

high-fat milk products
(whole milk, cream,
half-and-half,
chocolate milk, milk
shakes)

whole yogurt
any yogurt with stir-in
candies or sweetened
cereals
yogurts with aspartame

Fatty Foods

deep-fried foods (french
fries, fish, tempura,
doughnuts)

fast food (hamburgers,
hot dogs, fried pies)
any grilled meat

Spreads

margarine or oleo
butter substitutes

oil spreads
low-fat spreads

Artificial Sweeteners

aspartame
NutraSweet
Equal
saccharin

any food or drink
containing these
products

Fat Substitutes

Olestra
Simpless

any food or drink
containing these
products

Vegetable Oils and Saturated Fats

corn oil
soybean oil
lard

suet
vegetable shortening

22

Overweight Diet Plan

*I*f you are overweight but otherwise healthy, this is the diet plan you should try.

There is some evidence that being overweight may increase the chance of cancer recurrence, especially with hormonally related cancers. In breast cancer patients who are overweight, weight loss can aid the healing process.

Be realistic in setting goals. You do not have to aim for the often unrealistically low "desirable" weight. A moderate reduction of ten to twenty pounds has much the same benefits with less chance of regaining the lost weight and less stress on the body and mind. If your diet has differed significantly from the basic diet in Chapter 20, it may be more prudent to start there. If you do not lose one or two pounds in a month, switch to this diet.

The Diet Plan

This is a whole-foods diet designed to produce a slow and steady weight loss. It is high in vegetable protein and fiber and low in total fat and saturated fat. It emphasizes nutritionally dense foods such as beans, peas, lentils, vegetables, fruits, nuts, seeds, and food supplements to maintain lean muscle mass while decreasing fat stores.

Macronutrient Guidelines
- 20 percent calories from fat (from fish, poultry, flaxseed, fish oil, and olive oil)
- 55 percent calories from complex carbohydrate (from whole grains, legumes, and vegetables)
- 15 to 20 percent calories from protein (from beans, peas, and lentils)

- Eight to ten 8-ounce glasses of water each day (preferably filtered)

To know if you are consuming enough protein and calories, perform the following calculations:

Desirable weight: _____ pounds
   (See chart in chapter 20 and fill in your weight.)
Minimum daily protein requirement =
   Desirable weight × 0.5 = _____ grams
Daily calorie requirement (for men) =
   Desirable weight × 18 = _____ calories
Daily calorie requirement (for women) =
   Desirable weight × 16 = _____ calories

Meal Planning

- Eat five to six small meals rather than two to three large ones.
- If you cannot manage to eat all of the recommended vegetable servings, try juicing some of them. You can have up to sixteen ounces of vegetable juice a day.
- Foods that taste sweet should be eaten only with other foods.
- Cook meals that are appealing to the eye as well as the palate.
- Drink warm fluids such as soups and teas twenty minutes before meals.
- Drink eight to ten glasses of filtered water each day.
- Have plenty of vegetables and fruits on hand for snacks.
- Include protein-rich foods with meals.
- A high-fiber diet will help to keep blood sugar levels even, better controlling the appetite.
- Exercise according to your physician's instructions.

A sudden weight loss is not normal. If you lose more than

one to two pounds a week, increase the serving sizes. If the loss continues, see your doctor immediately.

Supplement Regime

Along with the foods recommended, take the following supplements each day:

- *Vitamin E*—Take 1,600 IU as mixed tocopherols. Get part from the multivitamin and the remainder from the antioxidant supplement.
- *Vitamin K*—Take this vitamin as part of a multivitamin supplement. Large doses of vitamin E require extra vitamin K.
- *Mixed carotenes*—Take 100,000 IU as mixed carotenes. Get part from the multivitamin and the remainder from the antioxidant supplement.
- *Multivitamin/mineral formula*—Take the "optimal" recommended dosage stated on the bottle.
- *Antioxidant formula*—This should contain vitamin C, vitamin E, beta-carotene and mixed carotenes, and selenium. Some comprehensive formulas also contain green tea extract and silymarin.
- *Fish oil (EPA)*—Take 1,000–1,600 milligrams EPA as fish oil. The amount of EPA per capsule and gram of fish oil differs depending on the source. Check the bottle for EPA levels.

Warning: When supplementing any fat-soluble vitamin or oil, you must also take a vitamin E supplement to protect against oxidation.

Foods to Eat Every Day

Include the minimum number of servings every day. Some days your average serving size will be smaller, and other days it will be larger. Remember, the *number* of servings is more important than the *size* of the servings.

Cruciferous Vegetables

at least 2 – 3 servings a day (One serving may be juiced.)

broccoli

brussels sprouts

cabbage

bok choy

kale

collard and mustard
   greens

cauliflower

Antioxidant Vegetables

at least 1 – 2 servings a day (One serving may be juiced.)

yams

sweet potatoes

carrots

spinach

tomatoes

bell peppers

asparagus

Green Leafy Vegetables

1 – 2 servings a day (One serving may be juiced.)

Swiss chard

dark green lettuces
   (green and red
   loose-leaf, romaine,
   butter)

escarole

chicory

dandelion greens

sprouts

sorrel

What Is One Serving?

These are the average serving sizes. If you cannot eat this amount of food when you are in therapy, decrease the size but not the number of servings. Variety of food is more important than quantity of food.

In the beginning, always measure your food. You may think you are using one cup, but it may be more or less.

Bread, Cereal, Rice, and Pasta

1 slice bread
1 ounce ready-to-eat cereal (Check labels: 1 ounce equals ¼ cup to 2 cups, depending on the cereal.)
½ cup cooked cereal, rice, or pasta
½ bagel or English muffin
3 or 4 plain crackers (small)

Vegetables

1 cup raw leafy vegetables
½ cup other vegetables, cooked or chopped raw
½ cup fresh vegetable juice

Fruit

1 medium apple, banana, orange, nectarine, or peach
½ cup chopped, cooked, or dried fruit
¾ cup fruit juice

Milk, Yogurt, and Cheese

1 cup milk or yogurt
1½ ounces natural cheese (a thin slice or 1-inch cube)

Poultry, Fish, Beans, Eggs, and Nuts

2–3 ounces cooked poultry or fish (about the size of a deck of cards)
1 cup cooked beans
1 egg
2 tablespoons nut butter
A handful of seeds or shelled nuts

Fats and Oils

2 teaspoons vegetable or nut oil
2 teaspoons butter
2 teaspoons mayonnaise
1 tablespoon oil- or mayonnaise-based salad dressing

Other Vegetables

1 serving a day

potatoes
rutabaga
turnips
beets
winter and summer
  squash
cucumbers
pumpkin
corn
green beans
wax beans
snow peas
sea vegetables (kelp,

kombu, wakame,
agar-agar, dulse,
carrageenan, nori,
and sea lettuce, or
supplement)
mushrooms (shiitake,
maitake, reishi, or
mushroom extract)
radishes
okra
kohlrabi
water chestnuts

Fruit

1 – 2 servings a day with meals, including 1 citrus (One serving may be juiced.)

citrus fruits (oranges,
  lemons, grapefruit,
  tangerines)
fresh fruits (bananas,
  plums, peaches,
  apricots, cherries,
  apples, berries,

cantaloupe, apricots,
  mango, papaya, pears,
  strawberries,
  watermelon)
dried fruit (figs, dates,
  raisins, prunes)
stewed fruit (applesauce)

Legumes

2 – 3 servings a day (This can include 1 of the soy food servings.)

Beans (soybeans, adzuki
  beans, lima beans,
  black beans, black-
  eyed peas, brown
  beans, pinto beans,
  red beans, fava beans,
kidney beans, navy
  beans, white beans,
  and chickpeas)
lentils and split peas
green peas

Soy Products

at least 1 – 2 servings a day

soymilk (regular, low-
  fat, nonfat, fortified,
  vanilla, chocolate, and
  carob)
tofu
tempeh
soy nuts
soy flour
soy grits
soy cheese
soybeans
miso

Grains

at least 6 – 11 servings a day

whole grains (amaranth,
  barley, buckwheat,
  corn, kamut, millet,
  oats, quinoa, brown
  rice, rye, spelt,
  triticale, wheat,
  wild rice)
whole-grain pasta,
breads, crackers,
  flours, unsalted
  air-popped popcorn
cereals (hot and cold
  with no added sugar)
brans (oat, rice, wheat)
germs (wheat, rice
  polish)

Dairy Products
at least 1 serving a day

yogurt (low-fat, nonfat,
   plain, flavored)
milk (nonfat and skim
   unflavored,

buttermilk,
   acidophilus, nonfat
   powdered or instant)
cottage cheese (nonfat)

Seasonings
use liberally

garlic, onions, leeks,
   and scallions (raw
   and cooked)
gingerroot (juiced, raw,
   brewed)
hot peppers (dried, raw,
   cooked)
rosemary

curry
cumin
basil
caraway seeds
cloves
tarragon
turmeric

Fats and Oils
up to 2 servings a day

canola oil
olive oil
nut oils (walnut,
   macadamia, almond)

salad dressings (canola
   oil mayonnaise,
   dressing made with
   olive or canola oil)

Beverages
as desired

tea (green, black)
herbal teas (any
   unsweetened)
filtered water
ginger tea

coffee substitutes
   (Cafix, Postum,
   Roma, chicory, or
   roasted barley drinks)
rice milk

Foods to Eat Weekly

Butter

2 – 3 servings a week

butter (salted, unsalted,
  whipped)

Dairy Products

2 – 3 times a week

cheese
low-fat cream cheese
sour cream

evaporated or condensed
  milk

Eggs

4 – 6 eggs a week

cooked eggs

Nuts and Seeds

3 – 4 servings a week

fresh nuts (almonds,
  Brazil nuts, cashews,
  filberts, pecans, pine
  nuts, pistachios,
  and walnuts)
fresh unseasoned seeds
  (pumpkin seeds,
  sesame seeds,
  sunflower seeds,

flaxseed)
nut and seed butters
  (tahini or sesame seed
  butter, walnut butter,
  almond butter,
  hazelnut butter,
  cashew butter, and
  sunflower butter)
nut milks (almond milk)

Poultry and Fish
3 – 5 servings a week

skinless fresh poultry
(turkey, chicken,
game hens)
cooked fish (especially

fatty fish such as
salmon, mackerel,
herring)

Peanuts
1 serving a week

roasted, fresh, unsalted
peanuts

peanut butter

Sweets
1 – 2 times a week

unrefined sweeteners
(grain syrups, maple
syrup, honey, and
Sucanat)
diluted fruit juices
(fresh, frozen,
bottled)
hard candies

chocolate
sweetened cocoa
frozen desserts (ice
milk, frozen yogurt,
sorbet, sherbet,
juice pops)
fruit spreads and
preserves

Note: Never eat sweets on an empty stomach. Always eat them as part of a meal.

Foods to Avoid
Coffee

caffeine-free coffee
regular coffee
instant coffee
flavored coffee

drip coffee
lattes and other espresso
drinks
iced coffee

Sweetened Drinks

all bottled or canned
  soft drinks
  (regular, diet, and
  caffeine-free)
bottled and canned
  iced teas
juice-flavored drinks

(such as Sunny
  Delight)
powdered instant drinks
  (such as sweetened
  or unsweetened
  Kool-Aid, lemonade)
canned juices

Candy

chocolate bars
granola bars

fruit roll-ups
chocolate-covered fruit

Smoked, Cured, or Pickled Foods

bacon
hot dogs
smoked luncheon meats
pepperoni and other
  smoked sausages
ham

Spam
canned meat spreads
pickled eggs
pickles
pickled herring

Meat

beef
buffalo
pork
ham
bacon

processed meats
liver
heart
tripe
pig's feet

Raw Animal Foods

raw or undercooked
  eggs
sushi (raw fish)

any other raw animal
  food

Refined or Processed Foods

white sugar

white-flour products
   (pancake mixes,
   cake mixes,
   pudding mixes)

refined cereals

white bread

cakes

pies

gelatins

prepared puddings

yogurts with candy
   stir-ins

Salty Foods

potato chips

corn chips

pretzels

theater-style popcorn

canned regular soups

high-sodium seasonings

any other salty food

Dairy Products

high-fat milk products
   (whole milk, cream,
   half-and-half,
   chocolate milk,
   milk shakes)

whole yogurt

any yogurt with stir-in
   candies or sweetened
   cereals

yogurt with aspartame

Fatty Foods

deep-fried foods
   (french fries, fish,
   tempura, doughnuts)

fast food (hamburgers,

hot dogs, fried pies,
   tacos, burritos)

any grilled meat

poultry skin

Alcohol

whiskey

rum

bourbon

tequila

gin

wine

beer

liqueurs

Spreads

margarine and oleo

butter substitutes

oil spreads

low-fat spreads

Artificial Sweeteners

aspartame

NutraSweet

Equal

saccharin

any food or drink

    containing these

    products

Fat Substitutes

Olestra

Simpless

any food or drink

    containing these

    products

Vegetable Oils and Saturated Fats

corn oil

soybean oil

lard

suet

vegetable shortening

23

Chemotherapy Diet Plan

During chemotherapy, the body is under stress. The guidelines in this chapter will help you give your body the resources it needs to cope.

Chemotherapy is recommended for patients whose cancers have the potential to spread, have spread, or are suspected of having spread to distant sites. Since chemotherapeutic agents are not limited to any particular area, they can circulate throughout your body, hopefully killing cancer cells that think they have escaped detection.

Many of the drugs used in chemotherapy interfere with cell division, because cancer cells divide faster than most normal tissue cells. When a drug interferes with cell division, the rapidly dividing cells are affected the most. This includes not only cancer cells, but the epithelial tissues that line the mouth, throat, and intestines. In the mouth, chemotherapy can cause mouth sores, tender or bleeding gums, sore throat, and difficulty swallowing. In the stomach it causes nausea and in the intestine, diarrhea.

The severity of chemotherapeutic side effects is related to the drug used, size of the dosage, length of treatment, and your individual response. Not everyone will have side effects. Some people breeze through the whole experience without giving it much thought. For others, chemotherapy becomes a full-time job.

Nutrition therapy during chemotherapy allows you to support healthy tissue while enhancing the toxicity to cancerous tissue. Cancer patients who have proper nutritional balance during chemotherapy have a better response and success rate with treatments.

Specific recommendations for nutritionally related side effects appear in Part II. Just add those dietary recommendations to the diet plan in this chapter.

The Diet Plan

This is a whole-foods diet high in vegetable protein and fiber and low in total fat and saturated fat. It is designed to support the body and minimize side effects while enhancing the ability of the chemotherapeutic agents to kill the cancer.

Macronutrient Guidelines
- 20 percent calories from fat (from fish, poultry, flaxseed, fish oil, and olive oil)
- 50 to 60 percent calories from complex carbohydrate (from whole grains, legumes, and vegetables)
- 20 to 30 percent calories from protein (from beans, peas, and lentils)
- Eight to ten 8-ounce glasses of water each day (preferably filtered)

To see if you are consuming enough protein and calories, perform the following calculations:

Desirable weight: _____ pounds
   (See chart in chapter 20 and fill in your weight.)
Minimum daily protein requirement =
   Desirable weight × 0.5 = _____ grams
Daily calorie requirement (for men) =
   Desirable weight × 18 = _____ calories
Daily calorie requirement (for women) =
   Desirable weight × 16 = _____ calories

Meal Planning
- Eat five to six small meals rather than two to three large ones.

- If you cannot manage to eat all of the recommended vegetable servings, try juicing some of them. You can have up to sixteen ounces of vegetable juice a day.
- Foods that taste sweet should be eaten only with other foods.
- Cook meals that are appealing to the eye as well as the palate.
- Drink eight to ten glasses of filtered water each day.
- Read the chapters on any side effects you experience.
- Always eat a protein-rich food with meals to keep blood sugar levels even, better controlling appetite.
- Exercise according to your physician's instructions.

If you lose more than a pound on this diet, increase serving sizes or add a handful of nuts or seeds. If the weight loss continues, notify your doctor immediately. Weight loss can be a sign of serious medical problems. A 5 percent weight loss from your normal weight is considered significant.

If you do not obtain enough calories, proteins, and nutrients from this whole-foods diet and do not gain and maintain the proper weight, a nutritional supplement may be necessary. We prefer homemade protein shakes and a multivitamin to the canned liquid supplements.

Supplement Regime for Chemotherapy

Along with the foods recommended, take the following supplements each day:

- *Vitamin E*—Take 1,600 IU as mixed tocopherols. Get part from the multivitamin and the remainder from the antioxidant supplement.
- *Vitamin K*—Take this vitamin as part of a multivitamin supplement. Large doses of vitamin E require extra vitamin K.
- *Mixed carotenes*—Take 100,000 IU as mixed carotenes. Get part from the multivitamin and the remainder from the antioxidant supplement.

- *Multivitamin/mineral formula*—Take the "optimal" recommended dosage stated on the bottle.
- *Antioxidant formula*—This should contain vitamin C, vitamin E, beta-carotene and mixed carotenes, and selenium. Some comprehensive formulas also contain green tea extract and silymarin.
- *Fish oil (epa)*—Take 1,000–1,600 milligrams EPA as fish oil. The amount of EPA per capsule and gram of fish oil differs depending on the source. Check the bottle for EPA levels.
- *Coenzyme Q_{10}*—Take 200 micrograms. Can be taken as part of a multivitamin supplement.
- *Cysteine or N-acetylcysteine*—Take one to two grams of this amino acid every eight hours.
- *Cruciferous vegetables*—Take four ounces of juice. This can be added to carrot juice or apple juice, or to soups or stews after cooking.
- *Rice bran*—Work up to 1 tablespoon a day.
- *Silymarin* (milk thistle seed extract)—Take 100 milligrams two to three times a day.
- *Green tea*—Drink one or two cups a day, or take green tea extract in capsule form.

Warning: When supplementing any fat-soluble vitamin or oil, you must also take a vitamin E supplement to protect against oxidation.

Foods to Eat Every Day

Include the minimum number of servings every day. Some days your average serving size will be smaller, and other days it will be larger. Remember, the *number* of servings is more important than the *size* of the servings.

Cruciferous Vegetables
at least 2 servings a day (One serving may be juiced.)

broccoli
brussels sprouts
cabbage
bok choy

kale
collard and mustard
   greens
cauliflower

Antioxidant Vegetables
at least 1 – 2 servings a day (One serving may be juiced.)

yams
sweet potatoes
carrots
spinach

tomatoes
bell peppers
asparagus

Green Leafy Vegetables
at least 1 – 2 servings a day

Swiss chard
dark green lettuces
   (green and red
   loose-leaf, romaine,
   butter)

escarole
chicory
dandelion greens
sprouts
sorrel

Nutrition Checklist for Chemotherapy

Before Treatment

☐ Vitamin E (1,600 IU) may help to prevent hair loss when taken seven to ten days before the start of therapy.

☐ Cystine, an amino acid, may help to protect healthy cells when taken seven to ten days before start of therapy.

☐ Glutathione may also help to protect cells when taken the week before treatment.

During Treatment

☐ Vitamin E, Vitamin A, and garlic may increase the effectiveness of chemotherapy.

☐ Bovine cartilage may prevent angiogenesis (new blood vessel growth), which is necessary for the tumor to grow and spread.

To Prevent or Slow Metastasis

☐ Fish oil as EPA and DHA which decreases the ability of cancer cells to stick.

☐ Fiber-rich foods keep blood sugar levels even. This will help to "starve" the glucose-hungry cancer cells.

☐ Eliminate sucrose, which may depress immune function.

To Protect Healthy Cells

☐ Vitamin C and the other antioxidant nutrients—selenium, vitamin E, and mixed carotenes—provide protection from the free radicals used to kill cancer cells (friendly fire). Take these as part of an antioxidant supplement.

☐ Coenzyme Q_{10} may protect the heart muscle from toxic drugs.

☐ Green tea contains strong antioxidants (and its tannins may prevent metastasis).

To Increase Detoxification of Chemotherapeutic Drugs

☐ Rice and wheat bran will increase the fecal excretion of drugs.

☐ Cruciferous vegetables will increase the production of the enzyme glutathione.

☐ N-acetylcysteine, an amino acid, will increase the enzyme glutathione.

☐ Silymarin (milk thistle seed extract) is well known for its ability to protect the liver from toxic chemicals.

Other Vegetables
at least 1 serving a day

potatoes
rutabaga
turnips
beets
winter and summer
   squash
cucumbers
pumpkin
corn
green beans
wax beans
snow peas
sea vegetables (kelp,

kombu, wakame,
agar-agar, dulse,
carrageenan, nori,
and sea lettuce, or
supplement)
mushrooms (shiitake,
maitake, reishi, or
mushroom extract)
radishes
okra
kohlrabi
water chestnuts

Fruit
at least 2 servings a day with meals, including 1 citrus (One serving may be juiced.)

citrus fruits (oranges,
   lemons, grapefruit,
   tangerines)
fresh fruits (bananas,
   plums, peaches,
   apricots, cherries,
   apples, berries,

cantaloupe, apricots,
   mango, papaya,
   pears, strawberries,
   watermelon)
dried fruit (figs, dates,
   raisins, prunes)
stewed fruit (applesauce)

Legumes

at least 2 servings a day (including 1 serving of soyfoods)

beans (soybeans, adzuki beans, lima beans, black beans, black-eyed peas, brown beans, pinto beans, red beans, fava beans, kidney beans, navy beans, white beans, and chickpeas)

lentils and split peas

green peas

Nuts and Seeds

at least 1 serving a day

fresh nuts (almonds, Brazil nuts, cashews, filberts, pecans, pine nuts, pistachios, and walnuts)

fresh unseasoned seeds (pumpkin seeds, sesame seeds, sunflower seeds, flaxseed)

nut and seed butters (tahini or sesame seed butter, walnut butter, almond butter, hazelnut butter, cashew butter, and sunflower butter)

nut milks (almond milk)

Soy Products

at least 1 – 2 servings a day

soymilk (regular, low-fat, nonfat, fortified, vanilla, chocolate, and carob)

tofu

tempeh

soy nuts

soy flour

soy grits

soy cheese

soybeans

miso

Grains
at least 6–11 servings a day

whole grains (amaranth, barley, buckwheat, corn, kamut, millet, oats, quinoa, brown rice, rye, spelt, triticale, wheat, wild rice)
whole-grain pasta,

breads, crackers, flours, unsalted air-popped popcorn
cereals (hot and cold with no added sugar)
brans (oat, rice, wheat)
germs (wheat, rice polish)

Dairy Products
at least 1 serving a day

yogurt (low-fat, nonfat, plain, flavored)
milk (nonfat and skim unflavored, buttermilk,

acidophilus, nonfat powdered or instant)
cottage cheese (nonfat, low-fat)

Seasonings
use liberally

garlic, onions, leeks, and scallions (raw and cooked)
gingerroot (juiced, raw, brewed)
hot peppers (dried, raw, cooked)
rosemary

curry
cumin
basil
caraway seeds
cloves
tarragon
turmeric

Fats and Oils
up to 2 servings a day

canola oil
olive oil
nut oils (walnut,
  macadamia, almond)

salad dressings (canola
  oil mayonnaise,
  dressings made with
  olive or canola oil)

Beverages
as desired

tea (green, black)
herbal teas (any
  unsweetened)
filtered water
ginger tea

coffee substitutes (Cafix,
  Postum, Roma,
  chicory, or roasted
  barley drinks)
rice milk

Food to Eat Weekly (Optional)

Butter
2–3 servings a week

butter (salted, unsalted,
  whipped)

Dairy Products
2–3 servings a week

cheese
low-fat cream cheese
low-fat sour cream

evaporated or condensed
  milk

Eggs
4–6 eggs a week

cooked eggs

Poultry and Fish

3 – 5 servings a week

skinless fresh poultry
(turkey, chicken,
game hens)
cooked fish (especially

fatty fish such as
salmon, mackerel,
herring)

Peanuts

1 serving a week

roasted, fresh, unsalted
peanuts

peanut butter

Note: Peanut butter is not recommended as an everyday food because of the normally high levels of aflatoxins present. Overconsumption of aflatoxins has been known to be carcinogenic. However, many other nut butters do not have high levels of aflatoxins.

Sweets

1 – 2 times a week

unrefined sweeteners
(grain syrups, maple
syrup, honey, and
Sucanat
diluted fruit juices
(fresh, frozen,
bottled)
hard candies

chocolate
sweetened cocoa
frozen desserts
(ice milk, frozen
yogurt, sorbet,
sherbet, juice pops)
fruit spreads and
preserves

Note: Never eat sweets on an empty stomach. Always eat them as part of a meal.

Foods to Avoid

Coffee

caffeine-free coffee
regular coffee
instant coffee
flavored coffee

drip coffee
lattes and other espresso
   drinks
iced coffee

Sweetened Drinks

all bottled or canned
   soft drinks
      (regular, diet, and
      caffeine-free)
bottled and canned
   iced teas
juice-flavored drinks

(such as Sunny
   Delight)
powdered instant drinks
   (such as sweetened
   or unsweetened
   Kool-Aid, lemonade)
canned juices

Candy

candy bars
granola bars

fruit roll-ups
chocolate-covered fruit

Smoked, Cured, or Pickled Foods

bacon
hot dogs
smoked luncheon meats
pepperoni and other
   smoked sausages
ham

Spam
canned meat spreads
pickled eggs
pickles
pickled herring

Meat

beef
buffalo
pork
ham
bacon

processed meats
liver
heart
tripe
pig's feet

Raw Animal Foods

raw or undercooked
    eggs
sushi (raw fish)

any other raw animal
    food

Refined or Processed Foods

white sugar
white-flour products
    (pancake mixes, cake
    mixes, pudding
    mixes)
refined cereals

white bread
cakes
pies
gelatins
prepared puddings

Salty Foods

potato chips
corn chips
pretzels
theater-style popcorn

canned regular soups
high-sodium seasonings
any other salty food

Dairy Products

high-fat milk products
    (whole milk, cream,
    half-and-half,
    chocolate milk, milk
    shakes)

whole yogurt
any yogurt with stir-in
    candies or sweetened
    cereals
yogurt with aspartame

Fatty Foods

deep-fried foods (french
    fries, fish, tempura,
    doughnuts)
fast food (hamburgers,

    hot dogs, fried pies)
any grilled meat
poultry skin

Alcohol

whiskey
rum
bourbon
tequila

gin
wine
beer
liqueurs

Spreads

margarine and oleo   oil spreads
butter substitutes   low-fat spreads

Artificial Sweeteners

Aspartame   any food or drink
NutraSweet   containing these
Equal   products
saccharin

Fat Substitutes

Olestra   any food or drink
Simpless   containing these
                                products

Vegetable Oils and Saturated Fats

corn oil   suet
soybean oil   vegetable shortening
lard

Nutrition-Related Side Effects of Chemotherapeutic Drugs

Alkylating Agents

busulfan
chlorambucil
cyclophosphamide
dacarbazine
ifosfamide
mechlorethamine
melphalan
streptozocin
thiotepa

Alkylating agents are used in the treatment of chronic leukemias, Hodgkin's disease, lymphomas, and some cancers of the lung, breast, prostate, and ovary. They work by substituting an alkyl group for a hydrogen atom. They are cell cycle phase nonspecific, which means they do not act on cells during any specific phase of cell division. These drugs work by interfering with DNA replication and RNA transcription.

Nutritional Side Effects

Nausea, vomiting, sore mouth and throat, sores on tongue or other areas of mouth and throat, bladder inflammation.

Nutritional Coping Strategies

Drink extra fluids to prevent kidney and bladder problems.

Nitrosoureas

carmustine
lomustine
semustine

Nitrosoureas cross the blood-brain barrier and are often used to treat brain tumors, lymphomas, multiple mylenomas, and malignant melanoma. These agents have a similar action to alkylating agents, as well as inhibiting the enzymes that repair DNA.

Nutritional Side Effects

Nausea, vomiting, sore mouth and throat, sores on tongue or other areas of mouth and throat, bladder inflammation.

Nutritional Coping Strategies

Drink extra fluids to prevent kidney and bladder problems.

Antibiotics

bleomycin
dactinomycin
daunorubicin
doxorubicin
mitoxantrone
mitomycin-C
plicamycin

Antibiotics are used to treat a wide variety of malignancies. They are used to kill cancer cells in much the same way they kill bacteria, by preventing cell division. This is done by binding to DNA and interfering with RNA transcription.

Nutritional Side Effects

Nausea; vomiting; inflammation of the mucous membranes; sores on the tongue, mouth, or throat; gastrointestinal upset.

Some antibiotics may decrease calcium and iron absorption.

Nutritional Coping Strategies

Drink extra fluids to prevent kidney and bladder problems.

Antimetabolites

cytarabine
methotrexate
5-fluorodeoxyuridine
5-fluorouracil
6-mercaptopurine
6-thioguanine

Antimetabolites may be used in the treatment of acute and chronic leukemias, choriocarcinoma, and some cancers of the gastrointestinal tract, breast, and ovary. They are substituted for purines or pyrimidines, necessary for normal cell division. Although these drugs fit into the spaces provided, they do not work once they are in.

Nutritional Side Effects

Nausea, vomiting, diarrhea, damage to the liver, inflammation of the mucous membranes.

Methotrexate acts as a folate antagonist and may decrease absorption of vitamin B_{12}, fat, and xylose.

Nutritional Coping Strategies

Drink extra fluids to prevent kidney and bladder problems. Avoid alcohol, which may increase the toxic effects of this drug, causing liver damage.

Hormones

diethylstilbestrol
fluoxymesterone
megestrol
acetate
prednisone
tamoxifen

Hormones are not toxic to cancer cells, so they are used to prevent further cell division and growth of hormone-dependent tumors. They work by changing the hormonal environment, making it unfriendly for tumor growth.

Nutritional Side Effects

Increased appetite, sodium and fluid retention, gastro-intestinal upset, glucose intolerance, potassium wasting, osteoporosis, negative nitrogen balance, loss of appetite, hypercalcemia, vomiting.

Nutritional Coping Strategies

If you take prednisone for a prolonged period, your doctor may want you to eat a potassium-rich diet. This drug may also decrease the effectiveness of insulin and other diabetic drugs.

Heavy Metals

cisplatin
carboplatin
Heavy metals cause cross-linking of DNA strands, which inhibits DNA synthesis.

Nutritional Side Effects

Nausea, vomiting, kidney toxicity, and low serum levels of magnesium, calcium, and zinc.

Plant (Vinca) Alkaloids

vinblastine
vincristine
etoposide
VP-16
Plant alkaloids are commonly used to treat acute lymphoblastic leukemia, Hodgkin's and non-Hodgkin's lymphomas, neuroblastomas, Wilms' tumor, and cancers of the lung, breast, and testes. They block cell division by not allowing spindle formation.

Nutritional Side Effects

Nausea, vomiting, constipation, and stomach cramps.

Nutritional Coping Strategies

Drink extra fluids to prevent kidney and bladder problems.

Enzymes

asparaginase
pegaspargase
Enzymes inhibit protein synthesis by depriving cells of asparagine.

Nutritional Side Effects

Nausea, vomiting, hypoalbuminemia (low albumin content of the blood), high blood sugar, inflammation of the pancreas, weight loss, stomach cramps, and uremia (buildup of uremic acid in the blood).

Nutritional Coping Strategies

Drink extra fluids to prevent kidney and bladder problems.

Biologic Response Modifiers

interferon
interleukin

Biological agents such as interferon and interleukin are used in patients with advanced cancer or cancer that has not responded to standard therapy. They destroy tumor cells by modifying the host's response to the tumor. They arm the immune army with weapons specific for cancer.

Nutritional Side Effects

Nausea, vomiting, loss of appetite, and weight change (up or down).

Nutritional Coping Strategies

Drink extra fluids to prevent kidney and bladder problems.

24

....

Radiation Therapy
Diet Plan

*B*ecause of the side effects of radiation therapy, people undergoing such treatment should follow this diet to give the body extra protection and strength.

Radiation therapy is used to treat localized tumors such as cancers of the skin, tongue, larynx, brain, breast, and cervix. Treatment exposes a defined area of tissue to ionizing radiation, damaging the DNA of all cells it reaches. The cancerous cells die from the injuries, but most normal cells will be able to repair themselves.

Gamma rays and x-rays are the two forms of photon energy used in **external radiotherapy**. They both have the same effect on cells and the same side effects. Cancerous cells can also be exposed to radiation using the technique of **internal radiotherapy**. Here radioactive implants are placed inside a tumor or body cavity. Internal radiation is often used for cancers of the tongue, uterus, and cervix. Radiation therapy can be used alone or in combination with chemotherapy or surgery.

Nutritional therapy during radiation therapy keeps the body nourished when side effects diminish appetite, protects the healthy cells from the effects of the radiation, makes the cancerous cells more vulnerable to the radiation, and speeds the healing of tissues damaged by radiation.

Radiation treatment can cause damage to the lining of the intestines, resulting in an inability to properly absorb protein, carbohydrate, fat, and other nutrients, as well loss of fluids and electrolytes. Add the specific recommendation for nutritionally related side effects from Part II to the diet plan found in this chapter.

The Diet Plan

This is a whole-foods diet high in vegetable protein and fiber and low in total fat and saturated fat. It emphasizes nutritionally dense foods such as beans, peas, lentils, vegetables, fruits, nuts, seeds, and food supplements to increase nutrient stores, strengthen the immune system, and weaken the tumor before radiation treatment begins.

Macronutrient Guidelines
- 20 percent fat (from fish, poultry, flaxseed, fish oil, and olive oil)
- 50 to 60 percent complex carbohydrate (from whole grains, legumes, and vegetables)
- 20 to 30 percent protein (from beans, peas, and lentils)
- Eight to ten 8-ounce glasses of water each day (preferably filtered)

To see if you are consuming enough protein and calories, perform the following calculations:

Desirable weight: _____ pounds
(See chart in chapter 20 and fill in your weight.)
Minimum daily protein requirement =
Desirable weight × 0.5 = _____ grams
Daily calorie requirement (for men) =
Desirable weight × 18 = _____ calories
Daily calorie requirement (for women) =
Desirable weight × 16 = _____ calories

Meal Planning

- Eat five to six small meals rather than two to three large ones.
- If you cannot manage to eat all of the recommended vegetable servings, try juicing some of them.
- Foods that taste sweet should be eaten only on a full stomach.
- Cook meals that are appealing to the eye as well as the palate.
- Drink eight to ten glasses of water (preferably filtered) a day.
- Read the chapter on any side effects you may be experiencing.
- Don't drink fluids or soups before or with meals. They will fill you up and leave no room for foods that are nutrient dense.
- Make mealtimes a pleasant experience by relaxing before the meal, eating with friends or family, and creating a pleasant atmosphere at the table.
- If you do not gain weight, increase serving sizes. If this does not work, notify your physician immediately. Loss of weight can be caused by serious medical problems.
- Radiation treatment to the abdomen can cause a temporary inability to digest lactose. A lactose-free diet plan appears in the next chapter.
- Radiation treatment to the abdomen can cause difficulty in digestion and absorption. Reduce raw fruits and vegetables and grain germs and brans.

If you do not obtain enough calories, proteins, and nutrients from this whole-foods diet and do not gain and maintain the proper weight, a nutritional supplement may be necessary. We prefer homemade protein shakes and a multivitamin to the canned liquid supplements.

Supplement Regime for Radiation Therapy

Along with the foods rocommended, take the following supplements each day:

- *Shark oil (alkylglycerols)*—Take two capsules per day, starting two weeks *before* treatment.
- *Multivitamin/mineral formula*—Take the "optimal" recommended dosage stated on the bottle. A recommended formula apears in the Appendixes at the end of this book.
- *Antioxidant formula*—This should contain vitamin C, vitamin E, beta-carotene and mixed carotenes, and selenium. Some comprehensive formulas also contain green tea extract and silymarin.
- *Mixed carotenes*—Take 100,000 IU as mixed carotenes. Get part from the multivitamin and the remainder from the antioxidant supplement.
- *Vitamin E*—Take 1,600 IU as mixed tocopherols. Get part from the multivitamin and the remainder from the antioxidant supplement.
- *Vitamin K*—Take this vitamin as part of a multivitamin supplement. Large doses of vitamin E require extra vitamin K.
- *Fish oil (EPA)*—Take 1,000–1,600 milligrams EPA as fish oil. The amount of EPA per capsule and gram of fish oil differs depending on the source. Check the bottle for EPA levels.
- *Vitamin B complex*—Take 50 milligrams B complex, sometimes called B-50.
- *Leafy green juice*—Take four ounces. This can be added to carrot juice, protein shakes, soups, and stews.
- *Glutamine*—Take two to four grams.
- *Vitamin B_6 as pyridoxal 5 pyrophosphate*—Take a total of 300 milligrams per day. Get part from the B complex supplement and part from the multivitamin/mineral

supplement; any remaining can be taken as a pure supplement.

- *Niacin as nicotinamide*—Take as part of the B complex supplement or the multivitamin/mineral supplement.

Warning: When supplementing any fat-soluble vitamin or oil, you must also take a vitamin E supplement to protect against oxidation.

Nutrition Checklist for Radiation Therapy

☐ Shark oil (alkylglycerols) may enhance tumor regression.

☐ Glutamine may protect against radiation-induced enteritis.

☐ Vitamin B, niacin, Vitamin C, and the other antioxidant nutrients (selenium, vitamin E, and mixed carotenes) protect healthy cells from radiation damage.

☐ Vitamin C and leafy green vegetables make cancer cells more vulnerable to radiation. Eat at least of two servings of leafy green vegetables each day. These make good additions to juices.

Foods to Eat Every Day

Include the minimum number of servings every day. Some days your average serving size will be smaller, and other days it will be larger. Remember, the *number* of servings is more important than the *size* of the servings.

Cruciferous Vegetables
at least 2 servings a day (One serving may be juiced.)

broccoli	kale
brussels sprouts	collard and mustard
cabbage	greens
bok choy	cauliflower

Antioxidant Vegetables
at least 2 servings a day (One serving may be juiced.)

yams	tomatoes
sweet potatoes	bell peppers
carrots	asparagus
spinach	

Green Leafy Vegetables
at least 2 servings a day

Swiss chard	escarole
dark green lettuces	chicory
(green and red	dandelion greens
loose-leaf, romaine,	sprouts
butter)	sorrel

Other Vegetables
1 serving a day (optional)

potatoes	kombu, wakame,
rutabaga	agar-agar, dulse,
turnips	carrageenan, nori,
beets	and sea lettuce, or
winter and summer	supplement)
squash	mushrooms (shiitake,
cucumbers	maitake, reishi, or
pumpkin	mushroom extract)
corn	radishes
green beans	okra
wax beans	kohlrabi
snow peas	water chestnuts
sea vegetables (kelp,	

What Is One Serving?

These are the average serving sizes. If you cannot eat this amount of food when you are in therapy, decrease the size but not the number of servings. Variety of food is more important than quantity of food.

In the beginning, always measure your food. You may think you are using one cup, but it may be more or less.

Bread, Cereal, Rice, and Pasta

1 slice bread
1 ounce ready-to-eat cereal (Check labels: 1 ounce equals ¼ cup to 2 cups, depending on the cereal.)
½ cup cooked cereal, rice, or pasta
½ bagel or English muffin
3 or 4 plain crackers (small)

Vegetables

1 cup raw leafy vegetables
½ cup other vegetables, cooked or chopped raw
½ cup fresh vegetable juice

Fruit

1 medium apple, banana, orange, nectarine, or peach
½ cup chopped, cooked, or dried fruit
¾ cup fruit juice

Milk, Yogurt, and Cheese

1 cup milk or yogurt
1½ ounces natural cheese (a thin slice or 1-inch cube)

Poultry, Fish, Beans, Eggs, and Nuts

2–3 ounces cooked poultry or fish (about the size of a deck of cards)
1 cup cooked beans
1 egg
2 tablespoons nut butter
A handful of seeds or shelled nuts

Fats and Oils

2 teaspoons vegetable or nut oil
2 teaspoons butter
2 teaspoons mayonnaise
1 tablespoon oil- or mayonnaise-based salad dressing

Fruit

at least 2 servings a day with meals, including 1 citrus (One serving may be juiced.)

citrus fruits (oranges, lemons, grapefruit, tangerines)
fresh fruits (bananas, plums, peaches, apricots, cherries, apples, berries, cantaloupe, mango, papaya, pears, strawberries, watermelon)
dried fruit (figs, dates, raisins, prunes)
stewed fruit (applesauce)

Legumes

at least 2 servings a day

beans (soybeans, adzuki beans, lima beans, black beans, black-eyed peas, brown beans, pinto beans, red beans, fava beans, kidney beans, navy beans, white beans, and chickpeas)
lentils and split peas
green peas

Nuts and Seeds

at least 1 serving a day

fresh nuts (almonds, Brazil nuts, cashews, filberts, pecans, pine nuts, pistachios, and walnuts)
fresh unseasoned seeds (pumpkin seeds, sesame seeds, sunflower seeds, flaxseed)
nut and seed butters (tahini or sesame seed butter, walnut butter, almond butter, hazelnut butter, cashew butter, and sunflower butter)
nut milks (almond milk)

Soy Products

at least 1 – 2 servings a day

soymilk (regular, low-
fat, nonfat, fortified,
vanilla, chocolate,
and carob)
tofu
tempeh

soy nuts
soy flour
soy grits
soy cheese
soybeans
miso

Grains

at least 6 – 11 servings a day

whole grains (amaranth,
barley, buckwheat,
corn, kamut, millet,
oats, quinoa, brown
rice, rye, spelt,
triticale, wheat,
wild rice)
whole-grain pasta,

breads, crackers,
flours, unsalted
air-popped popcorn
cereals (hot and cold
with no added sugar)
brans (oat, rice, wheat)
germs (wheat, rice
polish)

Dairy Products

at least 1 serving a day (including 1 serving of yogurt)

yogurt (low-fat, nonfat,
plain, flavored)
milk (nonfat and skim
unflavored,
buttermilk,

acidophilus, nonfat
powdered or instant)
cottage cheese (nonfat,
low-fat)

Seasonings
use liberally

garlic   rosemary
onions   curry
leeks   cumin
scallions (raw and   basil
   cooked)   caraway seeds
gingerroot (juiced, raw,   cloves
   brewed)   tarragon
hot peppers (dried, raw,   turmeric
   cooked)

Fats and Oils
up to 2 servings a day

canola oil   salad dressings (canola
olive oil   oil mayonnaise,
nut oils (walnut,   dressings made with
   macadamia, almond)   olive or canola oil)

Beverages
as desired

tea (green, black)   coffee substitutes
herbal teas (any   (Cafix, Postum,
   unsweetened)   Roma, chicory, or
filtered water   roasted barley drinks)
ginger tea   rice milk

Foods to Eat Weekly (Optional)

Butter
2–3 servings a week

butter (salted, unsalted,
   whipped)

Eggs

4–6 eggs a week

cooked eggs

Poultry and Fish

3–5 servings a week

skinless fresh poultry
(turkey, chicken,
game hens)
cooked fish (especially

fatty fish such as
salmon, mackerel,
herring)

Peanuts

1 serving a week

roasted, fresh, unsalted
peanuts

peanut butter

Note: Peanut butter is not recommended as an everyday food because of the normally high levels of aflatoxins present. Over-consumption of aflatoxins has been known to be carcinogenic. However, many other nut butters do not have high levels of aflatoxins.

Sweets

1–2 times a week

unrefined sweeteners
(grain syrups,
maple syrup, honey,
and Sucanat)
diluted fruit juices
(fresh, frozen,
bottled)
hard candies

chocolate
sweetened cocoa
frozen desserts
(ice milk, frozen
yogurt, sorbet,
sherbet, juice pops)
fruit spreads and
preserves

Note: Never eat sweets on an empty stomach. Always eat them as part of a meal.

Dairy Products
2 – 3 servings a week

cheese

low-fat cream cheese

sour cream

evaporated or condensed
  milk

Foods to Avoid

Coffee

caffeine-free coffee

regular coffee

instant coffee

flavored coffee

drip coffee

lattes and other espresso
  drinks

iced coffee

Sweetened Drinks

all bottled or
  canned soft drinks
  (regular, diet, and
  caffeine-free)

bottled and canned
  iced teas

juice-flavored drinks

(such as Sunny
  Delight)

powdered instant drinks
  (such as sweetened
  or unsweetened
  Kool-Aid, lemonade)

canned juices

Candy

candy bars

granola bars

fruit roll-ups

chocolate-covered fruit

Smoked, Cured, or Pickled Foods

bacon

hot dogs

smoked luncheon meats

pepperoni and other
  smoked sausages

ham

Spam

canned meat spreads

pickled eggs

pickles

pickled herring

Meat

beef	processed meats
buffalo	liver
pork	heart
ham	tripe
bacon	pig's feet

Raw Animal Foods

raw or undercooked eggs	any other raw animal food
sushi (raw fish)	

Refined or Processed Foods

white sugar	white bread
white-flour products (pancake mixes, cake mixes, pudding mixes)	cakes
	pies
	gelatins
	prepared puddings
refined cereals	

Salty Foods

potato chips	canned regular soups
corn chips	high-sodium seasonings
pretzels	any other salty food
theater-style popcorn	

Dairy Products

high-fat milk products (whole milk, cream, half-and-half, chocolate milk, milk shakes)	whole yogurt
	any yogurt with stir-in candies or sweetened cereals
	yogurt with aspartame

Fatty Foods

deep-fried foods
(french fries, fish,
tempura, doughnuts)
fast food (hamburgers,
hot dogs, fried pies)
any grilled meat
poultry skin

Alcohol

whiskey
rum
bourbon
tequila
gin
wine
beer
liqueurs

Spreads

margarine and oleo
butter substitutes
oil spreads
low-fat spreads

Artificial Sweeteners

aspartame
NutraSweet
Equal
saccharin
any food or drink
containing these
products

Fat Substitutes

Olestra
Simpless
any food or drink
containing these
products

Vegetable Oils and Saturated Fats

corn oil
soybean oil
lard
suet
vegetable shortening

25

Lactose-Free Diet Plan

*I*f you have trouble digesting dairy products, read this chapter for guidelines on how to modify your diet.

Lactose is the sugar found in milk and milk products. It is digested in the small intestine by the enzyme **lactase**, which lies on top of the intestinal villi. When the amount of lactase is reduced or not present at all, the milk sugar is not digested and passes untouched into the colon. There, the undigested sugar pulls water into the colon, causing cramps and diarrhea. Some of the lactose becomes dinner for the myriad of colonic bacteria, producing painful gas as an end product.

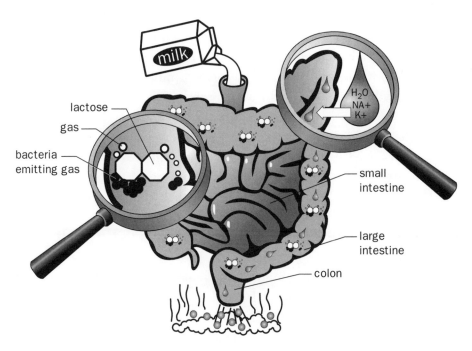

Lactose intolerance

Lactose Red Flags

When you see these words or ingredients on the label, the product probably contains lactose. This is another reason for avoiding processed, packaged foods during treatment. You can't always know for certain what you are eating.

Descriptions	*Ingredients*
Breaded	Breadings
Butter-flavored, buttery	Butter, butter solids
Cheese	Butter sauce
Chocolate flavored, chocolaty	Cheese solids
Chowder	Chocolate
Creamy, creamed	Cocoa
Milk	Milk
Pie	Milk solids
Sauce	Stuffing
Stuffed	Yogurt, yogurt solids

Do not confuse lactose intolerance with a milk allergy. Allergies are immune reactions to the *protein* in milk, whereas lactose intolerance involves the *sugar* in milk. Avoiding lactose will do you no good if your problem is a milk allergy.

As many as 30 million people in the United States lack sufficient quantities of lactase. But even those who have never experienced lactose intolerance before will have difficulty digesting dairy products during and after cancer treatments. This is the result of damage to the intestinal villi and the corresponding loss of the enzymes that lie on top of them. The condition is often temporary and fixes itself as the intestinal villi regrow.

If the intolerance is mild, you may simply need to supplement the missing enzyme, lactase, when you eat or drink a milk-containing product. This enzyme is available from two different companies in pill, liquid, and capsule forms. Pretreated lactose-reduced milk and lactose-free milk also are available.

For more severe or persistent symptoms, eliminate lactose from your diet. The remainder of this chapter explains how.

The Diet Plan

You can eat everything listed in the basic diet plan (Chapter 20) *except* the following foods and beverages:

- *Milk*—Avoid milk from all species, including goat, cow, and human milk; skim, nonfat, 1 percent, 2 percent, and whole milk; powdered, dried, and instant nonfat or low-fat milk; acidophilus milk, buttermilk, yogurt, and any other cultured milk product; chocolate and other flavored milks; hot chocolate and cocoa; evaporated or condensed milk; half-and-half; and whipped cream, whipping cream, and clotted cream.

- *Milk Products*—Do not eat or drink milk products, including low-fat, nonfat, and gourmet ice creams; ice milk, sherbet, frozen yogurt; milk shakes, and malts; milk puddings; sour cream; butter and margarine; chocolate and cocoa; and yogurt–fruit juice beverages.

- *Cheese*—Do not eat any cheese, including all types of natural cheese, cream cheese, cottage cheese, processed cheese, artificial and fat-free cheeses, and cheese cake.

- *Any other products that contain lactose*—To identify these products, read the ingredient label. Among the products that often contain lactose are flavored coffee mixes; some nondairy creamers; Ovaltine; creamed vegetables and vegetables in butter or cream sauces; creamed soups; some sauces, such as white, hollandaise, cheese, or cream; chowders; some breads, muffins, cookies, and other bakery items; some candies, such as toffee, butterscotch, caramels, fudge, and chocolates; dessert toppings such as chocolate syrup and hot fudge; desserts or entrees with a piecrust; French toast; some highly processed breakfast cereals, such as Total and Special K; flavored popcorns; omelets, soufflés, and quiches made with milk; some vitamins, food supplements, and medicines; and powdered sugar replacements such as Equal and Sweet'n Low.

Lactose-free milk and milk products are available. This will be marked on the label. You may find that taking an enzyme replacement before eating or drinking a lactose-containing food is all you need to do to avoid symptoms. Ask for lactose-free products at your local supermarket or health food store. You may also use one of the following milk substitutes.

These terms on a label indicate ingredients or foods that do not contain lactose:

- Any product marked "lactose free"
- Any product marked "pareve"
- Lactic acid
- Lactate
- Lactoalbumin
- Fortified soymilk
- Nut milks such as cashew milk or almond milk
- Rice milks such as Rice Dream

26

....

High-Fat Diet Plan

*I*f during treatment you have lost a lot of weight, your physician may want you to increase the amount of fats in your diet. If so, this chapter provides a diet plan that can help you.

Fats and other lipids are a concentrated source of energy. Carbohydrates and proteins each contribute four calories for every gram consumed. Fats contribute nine calories per gram, more than double the other energy sources. Fats are also easily stored in the body, providing you with a backup source of energy for times when you cannot eat.

We suggest that these fats be high in the monounsaturated fatty acids or those high in omega-3 fatty acids. Polyunsaturates have been shown in animal and human studies to speed tumor growth, and the sources of animal fats will tend to make your bodily fluids more acid, which is more hospitable for tumor growth. The fatty acids found in coconut milk are high in medium-chain triglycerides, which are easily absorbed with minimal digestion.

The high-fat foods in this diet plan will not only increase your calorie intake but will also aid in preventing metastasis and enhance the immune system. Add these foods to the underweight diet plan (Chapter 21) two servings at a time until the weight loss stops. Keep salted foods to a minimum. Salt can cause your body to hold water, and water weight can be mistaken for lean muscle weight gain.

Sometimes radiation and chemotherapy cause temporary intestinal damage, which decreases your ability to digest fats. If this happens your stools will be frequent, bulky, and light in color, a condition called steatorrhea. Sometimes treatment affects the liver's ability to produce bile, which also results in fat malabsorption. Pancreatic enzymes may also be reduced by treatment.

If you suffer from malabsorption, we strongly suggest that you take a digestive enzyme supplement. You will find a sample formula in the appendixes at the end of this book, along with the names of suppliers.

How Much Fat?

Each serving in the following list contains five grams of fat, which adds 45 calories to the diet. Thus, if you add four of these servings to the underweight diet plan (Chapter 21), you will obtain an additional 20 fat grams or 180 fat calories.

2 whole walnuts	1 tablespoon cashews
2 whole pecans	2–3 whole macadamia nuts
20 small peanuts	2 teaspoons peanut butter
10 small or 5 large olives	⅛ medium avocado
1 tablespoon pine nuts	1 tablespoon sunflower seeds
2 teaspoons pumpkin seeds	2 teaspoons tahini (sesame seed butter)
1 teaspoon olive, canola, safflower, or fish oil	2 tablespoons salad dressing
2 teaspoons canola mayonnaise	2½ teaspoons coconut milk
2 tablespoons shredded coconut	2 fish oil capsules (1,000 grams each)
¼ cup hummus with olive oil	½ cup firm tofu
1 ounce cooked Atlantic mackerel	1 ounce cooked Pacific herring
1 ounce cooked sablefish	3 ounces cooked salmon
1 ounce cooked American shad	2 ounces cooked trout
3 ounces cooked whitefish	3 ounces cooked yellowtail
3 ounces canned mackerel with bone	1 egg

The Diet Plan

Nuts and Seeds

whole nuts and seeds	sunflower seed butter
sesame seed butter (tahini)	other nut and seed butters
hazelnut butter	coconut milk
peanut butter (actually a legume butter)	Amasake (almond milk) other nut milks

Nuts and seeds are rich in cancer-fighting oils. Avoid nuts and seeds that are flavored, oiled, fried, or salted. Eat yogurt or chocolate-coated nuts in small amounts.

Serving Suggestions: Sprinkle seeds and crushed nuts on cereals, vegetables, and salads. Mix them with a small amount of dried fruit and eat as a snack or small meal. Use them to add a crunchy topping to casseroles.

To make your own nut butter, just add fresh unsalted nuts to a blender, food processor, or food grinder. Add sweeteners such as molasses or honey and seasonings such as cinnamon or nutmeg. Process until smooth. Make savory nut butters by adding garlic, onions, peppers, or other seasonings to the unsweetened nuts. Dilute nut butters with one of the oils recommended for this diet plan. Use the diluted nut butter as a salad dressing or mix it with a little soymilk and use as a vegetable dip or sauce.

Nut milks can be purchased in your local health food store and some grocery stores, but you can easily make them at home. Add a handful of nuts to a blender with 1 cup of filtered water. Process until the water is milky in color. Strain to remove the fiber, and store in the refrigerator. Nut milks can be sweetened with honey or molasses, then blended with fruit juice, dried fruit, soft whole fruit, yogurt, or soymilk to produce a calorie-rich meal shake.

Oils

extra-virgin olive oil
cold-pressed canola oil
high-oleic safflower oil

salad dressings made
    with one of the above
mayonnaise made with
    one of the above

Other High-Fat Foods

avocado
guacamole

olives
eggs

Part IV
Appendixes

Glossary

aflatoxin A highly carcinogenic mold that grows on grains and legumes, peanuts in particular.

ageusia Complete loss of the ability to taste.

allergy An overreaction to an antigen in an amount that does not affect most people.

antibody One of millions of blood proteins, produced by the immune system, that specifically recognizes a foreign substance and initiates its removal from the body.

antigen Any substance that stimulates the production of an antibody or antibodies upon introduction into the body of a vertebrate.

anticipatory nausea An upset stomach before treatment caused by the thought of treatment or even the sight of the hospital or clinic where treatment is given.

antiemetics Drugs that reduce nausea and vomiting.

antihistamines Chemical substances that neutralize histamine. Vitamin C is a natural antihistamine.

antioxidants Substances that prevent oxidation or the removal of electrons from molecules.

benign Not cancerous.

B cell A type of lymphocyte involved in the cellular immune response. The final stages of its development occur in bone marrow.

bone marrow The inner spongy tissue of bones where blood cells are made.

cancer A general name for over 100 diseases in which abnormal cells grow out of control; a malignant tumor.

carcinogenic Capable of initiating malignant transformation.

carcinogenesis The multistep process by which a normal cell becomes malignant.

carcinoma A cancer that originates in the epithelial tissue.

chemotherapy The use of drugs to stop cancer cells from growing in size or number.

combination chemotherapy The use of more than one drug to treat cancer.

complement system A group of eleven proteins that play a role in some reactions of the immune system. The complement proteins are not immunoglobulins.

constipation Difficulty in defecation accompanied by the passing of hard, small stools.

colonic Having to do with the colon or large intestine.

cytotoxic Toxic or poisonous to certain cells.

cytotoxic T cells Cells of the cellular immune system that recognize and directly eliminate virus-infected cells. (Contrast with *helper T cells,* and *suppresser T cells.*)

defecation A reflex caused by stimulation of receptors in the lining of the rectum.

dehydration Loss of too much body water, causing the body to malfunction. Severe diarrhea or vomiting can cause dehydration.

diarrhea Watery stools.

diet The foods a person eats on a regular basis.

differentiation The process by which normal cells undergo physical and structural changes as they develop to form different tissues of the body.

diuretics Drugs that help the body get rid of excess water and salt.

dysgeusia A change in the sense of taste.

dysphagia Difficulty in swallowing.

edema Buildup of extra fluid in the body's tissues.

electrolytes A general term for the minerals responsible for proper fluid balance, including sodium, potassium, chloride, and calcium.

emesis Vomiting.

emetic center The area of the brain that controls vomiting.

emetogenic potential The ability of a drug to cause nausea and vomiting. Drugs such as cisplatin, dacarbazine, and mechlorethamine have a high emetogenic potential, since they cause nausea and vomiting in over 90 percent of patients.

enteritis Inflammation of the lining of the intestines.

food aversion A learned dislike of foods that were eaten close to the time of a nausea-causing treatment and therefore have become linked in the brain with the symptoms caused by the treatment. Aromatic foods are at greatest risk for this.

free radicals Destructive charged particles with an extra electron. They are highly unstable until they find another electron to pair with. Antioxidants provide this extra electron, which stabilizes free radicals.

glucose A monosaccharide, or sugar made up of one carbon ring; the form of sugar found in blood.

helper T cells T cells that participate in the activation of B cells and of other T cells. (Contrast with *cytotoxic T cells,* and *suppresser T cells.*)

hypogeusia A decrease in the ability to taste.

immunoglobulin A class of proteins that have a characteristic structure and are active as receptors and effectors in the immune system.

interleukins Regulatory proteins, produced by macrophages and lymphocytes, that act upon other lymphocytes and direct their development.

lactose The disaccharide, or double sugar, found in milk; also called milk sugar.

lactose intolerance Loss of the ability to digest lactose.

lymphocyte A major class of white blood cells; includes T cells, B cells, and other cell types important in the immune response.

macrophage A type of phagocytic white blood cell that patrols the tissues of the body.

malnutrition A state caused when the body does not receive essential nutrients.

metastasize Spread of a cancer tumor from the primary site to other locations in the body. Cancers tend to metastasize to specific organs or sites in the body.

malignant Cancerous.

mucositis An inflammation of the mucous membranes, causing mouth sores.

mutagenic Causing mutations or changes in DNA coding.

nausea Upset stomach.

nitrosamines A combination of amine and nitrous acid, which can be formed from nitrites in stomach acid. They are mutagenic or carcinogenic.

oncogenes Genes within the cell that may initiate the cell's transformation from normal to malignant.

peristalsis The contraction of intestinal muscles responsible for the movement of food through the gastrointestinal tract.

phagocyte A white blood cell that eats or engulfs microorganisms.

phytoestrogens Estrogen-like compounds found in plants.

saliva A mixture of secretions from the salivary and oral mucous glands that keeps the tissues of the mouth moist and lubricates food to facilitate swallowing.

salivary glands The glands that secrete saliva, including the large parotid, submaxillary, and sublingual glands.

sarcoma Cancers originating in the connective and muscle tissue.

sialagogue A drug or other agent that increases the flow of saliva.

staging The process of describing the extent of disease at the time of diagnosis in order to assess prognosis, aid in planning, treatment, and compare treatment approaches.

suppresser T cells T cells that inhibit the responses of B cells and other T cells to antigens. (Contrast with *cytotoxic T cells,* and *helper T cells.*)

synergistic Enhancing each other's effects. The whole is more powerful than the sum of the individual parts.

taste buds Chemical receptors for the taste nerve fibers.

T cell A type of lymphocyte, involved in the cellular immune response. The final stages of its development occur in the thymus gland. (Contrast with *B cell*; see also *cytotoxic T cell*, *helper T cell*, *suppresser T cell*.)

total parenteral nutrition (TPN) Receipt of all the nutrients the body needs through a needle in a vein. TPN is used when the mouth, stomach, or bowel is injured from cancer treatment.

tumor An abnormal growth, which may be either benign or malignant.

xerostomia A decrease in saliva that causes the sensation of a dry mouth.

yogurt bacteria The strains of *lactobacillus bulgaricus* and *Streptococcus thermophilus* or *Lactobacillus acidophilus* that are added to milk to make yogurt.

Sample Supplement Formulas

*T*ake these sample formulas to the health food store or to your health care professional. Choose a supplement that most closely resembles this formula.

Multivitamin/Multimineral Supplement

- Vitamin A (acetate), 10,000 IU
- Beta-carotene equivalent to 15,000 IU vitamin A
- Vitamin D_3 (cholecalciferol), 400 IU
- Vitamin E (d-alpha-tocopherol succinate), 400 IU
- Vitamin K_1 (phytonadione), 60 micrograms
- Vitamin C (ascorbic acid), 1,200 milligrams
- Vitamin B_1 (thiamine monotitrate), 28 milligrams
- Vitamin B_2 (riboflavin), 32 milligrams
- Vitamin B_3 (niacin), 20 milligrams
- Vitamin B_3 (niacinamide), 380 milligrams
- Pantothenic acid (calcium d-pantothenate), 150 milligrams
- Folic acid, 800 micrograms
- Vitamin B_{12}, 120 micrograms
- Dibencozide (vitamin B_{12} coenzyme), 500 micrograms
- Biotin, 300 micrograms
- Trimethylglycine HCl, 100 milligrams
- Choline (bitartrate), 125 milligrams
- Inositol, 120 milligrams
- PABA (para-aminobenzoic acid), 50 milligrams
- Bioflavonoids (undiluted), 100 milligrams
- Calcium (citrate, microcryctalline, hydroxyapatite, glycinate), 400 milligrams
- Magnesium (glycinate), 100 milligrams

- Potassium (aspartate), 99 milligrams
- Iron (glycinate), 10 milligrams
- Iodine (potassium iodide), 150 micrograms
- Chromium (nicotinate, glycinate), 200 micrograms
- Selenium (asparate), 100 micrograms
- Vanadyl sulfate, 200 micrograms
- Inosine, 80 milligrams
- Glutamine, 100 milligrams
- Copper (lysinate), 2 milligrams
- Zinc (glycinate, histidinate), 20 milligrams
- Manganese (glycinate), 8 milligrams

Individual Supplements

You may take individual supplements in doses up to the following amounts per day (instead of the preceding formulas):

- Vitamin A, 100,000 IU per day
- Vitamin B complex, 50 milligrams
- Vitamin C, 1,020 grams (take to bowel tolerance)
- Beta-carotene, 10,000 IU
- Vitamin E, 1,200 to 1,500 IU
- Zinc, 50 milligrams
- Co-Enzyme Q_{10}, generally 300 to 400 milligrams can be taken as high as 700 milligrams.
- Flaxseed oil, 1–2 tablespoons a day for three months and 1 tablespoon a day thereafter, or flaxseed capsules, 1,000 milligrams three times a day for three months and two times a day thereafter. Flaxseed oil and capsules provide omega-3 and omega-6 fatty acids, which are essential fatty acids. Other sources of essential fatty acids are borage oil, black currant oil, and primrose oil.

Resources for Patients and Families

Cancer Information Services (CIS) 1-800-CANCER
The CIS is a nationwide telephone service supported by the National Cancer Institute. Information specialists will provide information and publications on all aspects of cancer for patients and their families, health care professionals, and the general public. They may also be able to direct you to support groups and cancer services in your area.

American Cancer Society (ACS) 1-800-ACS-2345
The ACS is a nonprofit organization offering a variety of services to patients and their families. Programs to inquire about include the **CanSurmount Program**, a program that brings patients who have recovered from cancer together with newly diagnosed patients and patients whose cancer has recurred, to talk about cancer-related programs and treatments; and the **I CAN COPE Program**, a course designed to address the educational and psychological needs of people with cancer.

Reach to Recovery Program
National Coalition for Cancer Survivorship
(301) 650-8868
1010 Wayne Avenue
Silver Springs, MD 20910

Cancer Care Inc. 1-800-813-HOPE

The Wellness Community (310) 314-2555

YWCA of the USA's "Encore Plus" 1-800-958-PLUS
or (202) 628-3636

Amgen/Mediaworks video program (For Husbands and Friends) 1-800-333-9777 ext: 333

YMe (For Children) 1-800-221-2141

The Susan G. Komen Breast Cancer Foundation
1-800-462-9273 and (714) 380-4334

Product Descriptions
Multivitamins
Product: Multigenics (Intensive Care Formula (Multivitamin)
Manufacturer: Metagenics Corporation (1-800-338-3948)
Call to find out who sells these products in your area.

Product: ProGain
Manufacturer: Metagenics Corporation
(1-800-338-3948)
Description: ProGain is a high-nitrogen, high-calorie, di- and tripeptide liquid drink mix that provides many of the macro and micro nutrients necessary to promote weight gain, muscle mass, positive nitrogen balance, and energy enhancement. The combination of protein from purified lactoalbumin (enzymatically hydrolyzed) and carbohydrate from glucose polymers and pure, crystalline fructose results in optimal absorption, positive energy balance, and excellent tolerance for most people.

Enzymes
Product: Metazyme® NonAnimal Digestive Enzymes
Manufacturer: Metagenics Corporation
(1-800-338-3948)
Call to find out who sells these products in your area.

Product: Similase®
Manufacturer: Tyler Encapsulations (1-800-869-9705)
Call to find out who sells these products in your area.
Description: Highly concentrated digestive enzymes.

Product: Beano®
Description: Prevents flatulence from legumes and vegetables.

Product: Lactaid®
Description: An enzyme that digests lactose or milk sugar for those with permanent or temporary lactose intolerance.

Acidophilus Products
Manufacturer: Tyson (1-800-367-7744)
Manufacturer: Klair Labs (1-800-533-7255)
Manufacturer: Seraphim (1-800-525-7372)

Mail Order Resources
Bronson Corp.
1-800-235-3200
8 A.M. to 7 P.M. Central Standard Time
Bronson's vitamins and herbals are sold only through health professionals. Call for the names of those who are selling its products in your area. Products include black currant seed oil (essential fatty acids) with vitamin E, garlic capsules, lecithin granules, chewable digestive enzymes, and buffered powdered vitamin C.

Harvest Direct Inc.
Box 4514
Decatur, IL 62521-4514
1-800-835-2867
9 A.M. to 6 P.M. Eastern Standard Time
This company sells textured vegetable protein.

Health by Heidi
(415) 572-7100
This company sells green tea and green tea extract.

Metagenics Corporation
1-800-692-9400
1-800-338-3948
8 A.M. to 6 P.M. Pacific Standard Time
Metagenics supplements are sold only through health professionals. Call for the names of those who carry its products in your area. Products include vitamins and mineral combinations and a complete line of high-quality protein powders and enzymes.

Thorne Research, Inc.
1-800-228-1966
9 A.M. to 5 P.M. Pacific Standard Time
Thorne's vitamin, mineral, and encapsulated products are of high quality and are sold only through health professionals. Call for the names of those who carry its products in your area. Among Thorne's products appropriate for those undergoing cancer treatment are digestive enzymes, bioflavonoids, black currant oil, vitamins, minerals, and multivitamins.

Suggested Reading Materials

Books About Cancer

Breast Cancer: What You Should Know About Prevention, Diagnosis, and Treatment
by Dr. Steven Austin and Cathy Hitchcock
Prima Publishing, 1994
Rocklin, California

The Transformed Cell: Unlocking the Mysteries of Cancer
by Dr. Steven A. Rosenberg and John M. Barry
G. P. Putnam's Sons, 1992
New York, New York

Books on Nutrition

Beating Cancer with Nutrition
by Patrick Quillin with Noreen Quillin
The Nutrition Times Press, 1994
Tulsa, Oklahoma

Sharks Don't Get Cancer: How Shark Cartilage Could Save Your Life
by Dr. I. William Lane and Linda Comac
Avery Publishing Group Inc., 1992
Garden City Park, New York

Juicing for Good Health
by Maureen B. Keane
Pocket Books, 1992
Rocklin, California

Grains for Better Health
by Maureen B. Keane and Daniella Chace
Prima Publishing, 1994
Rocklin, California

Staying Healthy with Nutrition: The Complete Guide to Diet and Nutritional Medicine
by Dr. Elson M. Haas
Celestial Arts, 1992
Berkeley, California

The Healing Power of Herbs: The Enlightened Person's Guide to the Wonders of Medicinal Plants
by Dr. Michael Murray
Prima Publishing, 1991
Rocklin, California

The Encyclopedia of Natural Medicine
by Dr. Michael Murray and Dr. Joseph Pizzorno
Prima Publishing, 1990
Rocklin, California

Books for Professionals

Adjuvant Nutrition in Cancer Treatment:
1992 *Symposium Proceedings*
Edited by Patrick Quillin and Dr. Michael Williams
Cancer Treatment Research Foundation, 1994
Arlington Heights, Illinois

Nutritional Influences on Illness III
by Dr. Melvyn R. Werbach
Third Line Press Inc., 1995
Tarzana, California

Nutrition Treatment Plan

This dietary prescription is for:

Date:

Follow this diet:

☐ before treatment ☐ during treatment ☐ after treatment

☐ Normal diet ☐ Radiation diet
☐ Underweight diet ☐ High-fat diet
☐ Overweight diet ☐ Lactose-free diet
☐ Chemotherapy diet

Specific vitamins and food supplements/dosage/brand

-
-
-
-
-

These foods or food supplements could interfere with your therapy and should be avoided:

-
-

Additional dietary advice:

Specific dietary problems:

☐ Appetite loss ☐ Swallowing difficulties
☐ Constipation ☐ Taste changes
☐ Diarrhea ☐ Vomiting
☐ Dry mouth ☐ Upset stomach
☐ Mouth and throat sores

Read these sections:

☐ Dental Care ☐ Food preparation ☐ Lactose intolerance

Additional books to read:

Index

Leukocytes (white blood cells), 14
Libraries, 2
Lignin, 61–62
Linoleic acid, 72, 77, 97
Linolenic acid, 70, 72, 77
Lipases, 76
Lipids, 67, 73–78
and cancer, 77
compound, 74
function of, 75–76
metabolism of, 76–77
storage of, 75
types of, 73–74
Lipopolysaccharides, 74
Lipoproteins, 74
Liver, 31–32, 83, 89, 91, 98, 110, 116
Lobster, 107
Lomustine, 221
Low-density lipoprotein (LDL), 74
Lungs, 26–28, 112, 114
cancer of, 169, 221, 224
Lutein, 54, 110
Lycopene, 54, 110
Lymph, 24–26
Lymph nodes, 24–25
Lymph tissue, 51
Lymphatic system, 24–26, 76, 95
Lymphatic vessels, 24–26
Lymphocytes, 49–50, 91
Lymphokines, 51
Lymphomas, 11, 14, 26, 31, 221, 224
Lysosomes, 5

Mackerel, 90
Macro minerals, 100–103. *See also* Minerals; separate listings
Macronutrient guidelines
for basic diet, 160
for chemotherapy plan, 208
for overweight plan, 193–94
for radiation therapy plan, 228
for underweight plan, 180
Macrophages, 49, 96
Magnesium, 102
Malabsorption, 29, 30, 157
Maldigestion, 157
Malic acid, 105
Maltose, 58
Mangoes, 94
Margarines, 70. *See also* Spreads
Massage, 150

Matrix, 13
Mcts. *See* Medium-chain triglycerides
Meal planning
for basic diet, 160–62
for chemotherapy plan, 208–209
for overweight plan, 194–95
for radiation therapy plan, 229
for underweight plan, 180–81
Meals, 65, 128–29, 132. *See also* Diet plans; Food preparation; Meal planning
Meals on Wheels, 159
Meat, 175, 191, 203, 218, 239. *See also* individual listings
Mechlorethamine, 221
Mediastinum, 28
Medium-chain triglycerides (MCTS), 71, 76–77
Megadoses (vitamins), 89. *See also* Supplements
Megestrol, 223
Melanine, 96
Melanomas, 16, 19, 221
Melphalan, 221
Membrane, plasma, 4
Membranous epithelial tissues, 11–12
Menstruation, 105
Metastasis, 20, 32, 42, 98
Methionine, 82–83, 103
Methotrexate, 116, 136, 141, 222
Microvilli (intestinal), 29–30, 150
Milk, 71, 81, 83, 90, 92, 97, 129, 150, 152, 243
Millet, 90
Mineral balance, 96
Mineral deficiency, 99–100
Minerals, 20, 52, 99–107
Miso soup, 129
Mitimycin-C, 222
Mitochondria, 5
Mitosis, 6–8
Mitoxantrone, 222
Molasses, 93
Monocytes, 49
Monoglycerides, 73
Monosaccharides, 57–58
Monounsaturated fatty acid, 69
Mouth, 28–29, 131–33, 141–43. *See also* Oral health; Teeth

Mouthwash, 124
Mucinous adenocarcinomas, 23
Mucositis, 136, 141–43
Multivitamin formula. *See* Supplements
Mung beans, 90
Muscular system, 20–21
Muscles, 100, 102, 103
Mushroom extract, 166
Mushrooms, 90, 92, 113, 166
Mutation, genetic, 8
Myeloid cartilage, 14
Myeloma, multiple, 14
Mylenomas, 221
Myoglobin, 104
Myricetin, 54, 112

N-acetylcysteine, 210
Natural killer (NK) cells, 45, 50, 77, 96, 105, 106
Nausea, 113, 125–30
causes of, 127
severe, 130, 138
solutions for, 127–30
Neoplasia. *See* Tumors
Nephroblastoma, 33
Neuroglia cells, 15
Neurons (nerve cells), 15
Neuroblastomas, 224
Neurotransmitters, 21, 100
Neutrophils, 49
Nervous system, 21–22
Nervous tissue, 15–16, 148
cancers of, 11
Niacin, 82, 90–91, 231
Nitrogen, 84–85
Nitrogen balance, 84–85
Nitrosoureas, 221–22
NK cells. *See* Natural killer cells
Nonessential amino acids, 82
Nose, 26–27
Nucleus, cell, 4, 6
Nut butters, 129, 137, 217, 247
Nut milks, 247
Nutmeg, 113, 153
Nutrition, 30
chemistry of, 2
and immune system, 51–53
Nutrition checklists
for chemotherapy, 212
for radiation therapy, 231
Nuts, 84, 90, 98, 102, 106, 132, 149. *See also* separate listings

in diet plans, 168, 186,
201, 214, 234
serving suggestions for,
247

Oat bran, 148
Oatmeal, 92, 142, 152
Odor neutralizers, 129
Odors, 129, 135, 137,
139
Okra, 166
Oils, 67–70, 97, 129, 172
in diet plans, 172, 177,
188, 192, 200, 205,
216, 220, 236, 240,
248
hydrogenated, 69
polyunsaturated, 68–69
Omega number and
length, 70–71
Omega-6, 70–71, 77
Omega-3, 70, 85
Oncogenes, 169
Oncology, 41
Onions, 113, 129
Oral health, 123–24
Organ systems, 17–37
Organelles, 4
Orange juice, fortified,
102
Oranges, 110, 167
Organic produce, 159
Organosulfur compounds,
113
Ova, 35
Ovalbumin, 83
Ovaries, 22–23, 36, 110
cancer of, 221, 222
Overweight diet plan,
193–205
Oxidation, 97
Oysters, 104, 107

Painkillers, opioid, 147
Palate, 136
Pancreas, 22–23, 96, 100,
110
cancer of, 157
Pantothenic acid, 93, 102
Papaya, 94
Paprika, 111
Pap smear, 12
Parathyroid hormone, 97
Parenchyma, 43
Peaches, 110
Peanut butter, 129, 174,
217, 237
serving suggestions for,
174
Peanuts, 91, 174, 189, 202,
217, 237
Peas, 104

black-eyed, 92
split, 90, 92, 106, 152
Pegaspargase, 224
Penis, 35
Peppermint, 113, 129, 137
Peppers
hot, 129, 142
sweet, 94
Peptide bonds, 80–81
Peptide chains, 80
Peristalsis, 145, 149
Permeability, 111
PGE2. See Prostaglandin E2
series
Phagocytic cells, 49
Pharynx (throat), 26–27,
28–29
Phenothiazines, 90
Phenylalanine, 83
Phosphate groups, 6
Phosphates, 102
Phospholipids, 74
Phosphorus, 96, 100–102
absorption of, 101
Phytates, 102
Phytic acid, 104
Phytochemicals, 53, 85,
109–114
Phytoesterols, 114, 169
Pickled foods, 175, 191,
203, 218, 238
Pigment, 83, 96, 110, 111
Pineal gland, 22–23
Pine nuts, 91
Pituitary gland, 22–23
Placenta, 22–23
Plant protein, 84, 85
Plasma, blood, 14
Plasma membrane. See
Membrane, plasma
Plicamycin, 141, 222
Polypeptide chains, 80
Polysaccharides, 59–60
Portal system, 65
Potato chips, 129
Potatoes, 93, 104, 106,
142, 152, 166
Potassium, 103, 153
Poultry, 85, 92, 104, 105,
137, 174
in diet plans, 174, 189,
202, 217, 237
serving suggestions for,
174
Prednisone, 223
Pregnancy, 84, 91
Pressure-cooking, 121
Pretzels, 129
Primrose oil, 71, 77
Proanthocyanidins, 54
Processed foods, 91, 93,
105

in diet plans, 176, 191,
204, 219, 239
Progressive agents, 41
Promoters, 41
Prostaglandin E2 series
(PGE2), 71, 77, 112
Prostaglandins, 71
Prostate, 35, 112, 114
cancer of, 169, 221
Protease inhibitors, 114,
167, 169
Protein, 20–21, 53, 75,
79–85, 101
animal, 83
and cancer, 85
chemical composition of,
80–81
complete and
incomplete, 83–84
deficiency of, 84
fibrous, 80
globular, 81
sources of, 168, 169
Protein powders, 152
Prunes, 104, 150, 152
Pseudostratified columnar
epithelium, 12
Psyllium, 148
Pumpkin, 110, 166
Pyridoxal 5 pyrophosphate
(Vitamin B6), 230
Pyridoxine (Vitamin B6),
52, 88, 91
Pyrroloquinoline quinone,
88

Quercetin, 54, 112
Quinoa, 142, 149

Radiation therapy, 29, 30,
97, 105, 127
and diarrhea, 151
diet plan for, 227–40
and dry mouth, 131
and mucositis, 142
nutrition checklist for,
231
and taste alterations, 136
Radishes, 166
Raisins, 104
Rancidity (oils), 69, 97
Raw foods, 152, 176, 191,
203, 219, 239
RDA. See Recommended
Dietary Allowance
Receptor sites, 4
Recommended Dietary
Allowance (RDA), 88
Rectum, 28, 31, 112
Refined foods. See
Processed foods
Renal cell carcinoma, 33